I0359883

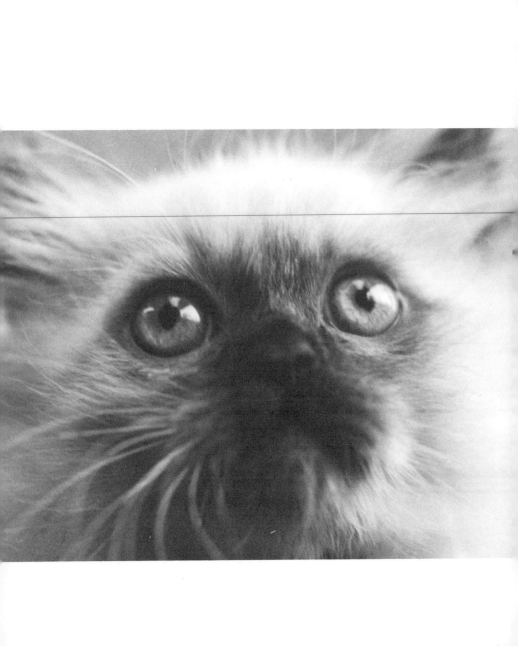

THE
WELL CAT
BOOK

THE
WELL CAT
BOOK

Terri McGinnis D.V.M.
Author Of The Well Dog Book

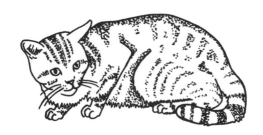

illustrated by
Tom Reed D.V.M.

A RANDOM HOUSE • BOOKWORKS BOOK

Copyright © 1975 by Terri McGinnis, D.V.M.
All rights reserved under International and
Pan American Copyright Conventions.

First printing, February 1975   12,500 copies in cloth
Second printing, June 1975   7,500 copies in cloth

Illustrations by Tom Reed, D.V.M.
Typeset by Vera Allen Composition Service, Hayward, California
   (With special thanks to Rosemay, Michele and Paul)
Printed and bound by Colonial Press, Clinton Massachusetts, under
the direction of Dean Ragland, Random House
Photos by John Pearson

This book is co-published by   Random House Inc
                               201 East 50th Street
                               New York N Y 10022

                            and The Bookworks
                               2043 Francisco Street
                               Berkeley California 94709

Distributed in the United States by Random House and simultaneously
published in Canada by Random House of Canada Ltd., Toronto.

Booksellers please order from Random House.

Library of Congress Cataloging in Publication Data

McGinnis, Terri
   The well cat book.

   "A Random House/Bookworks book."
   1. Cats–Diseases.   I. Title.
SF985.M32   636.8'08'96024   74-23050
ISBN 0-394-48946-2

Manufactured in the United States of America

For Louise,
who never seemed
to like cats much, but
couldn't keep me from
liking them.

How To Use This Book
For Quick Reference

TO UNDERSTAND
  your cat's body, turn to page 7.

TO FIND INFORMATION
  about daily cat care, turn to page 44.

FOR HELP DIAGNOSING
  the signs of illness or injury, turn to page 107.

IN AN EMERGENCY SITUATION,
  turn to page 168.

FOR HELP GIVING MEDICATION,
  turn to page 193.

FOR SOLUTIONS TO PROBLEMS
  of breeding and reproduction, turn to page 219.

Table of Contents

xiv

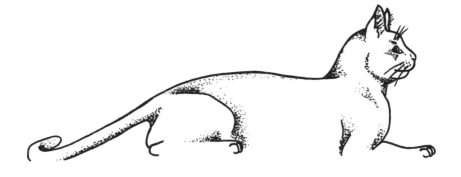

Introducing the Well Cat

The cat with which you share your home (or may be considering sharing it with) has a long and unclear history. Over thirty-five million years ago its first ancestors appeared. It is thought that they originated from a weasel-like meat-eater which was a member of an animal family called *Miacidae* (also thought to be ancestors of, among others, the dog, raccoon, bear, skunk and hyena). From these first cat ancestors arose two branches of recognizably cat-like creatures. One included the saber-toothed cats which eventually became extinct; the other included the ancestors of all the *Felidae* (cat family) alive today. Exactly when the cat became man's companion is not known. It is well documented, however, that cats closely resembling those alive today were an important part of the Egyptian culture (where they were revered and considered sacred) as early as 2500 B.C. From Egypt it appears that domestic cats were disseminated to the Far East and Europe and, much later (around the seventeenth century), imported to North America from Europe. Although the cat was condemned as a symbol of evil during the Middle Ages in Europe and at the time of the witch hunts in North America, for most of its history the cat has maintained its position as an important companion to man (perhaps because of its skill as a vermin killer). In fact, the cat has gained steadily in popularity and numbers since the 1700's until today in developed countries only the dog competes seriously with it for the public's affection. Over 28 million cats reside in the United States alone!

1

Although cats have been companions for so long, it is only within the last twenty-five years or so that veterinarians and cat owners have become interested in and able to provide very specialized health care for them. Some pet owners may want to step back and allow the veterinarian to solve any health problem their cat may have, but many are interested in taking an active part in preserving and maintaining their cat's good health. This book is written as a guide for those who wish to assume the primary responsibility for their cat's health and who want to pursue home treatment of it when possible.

The Well Cat Book differs from other books on cat care because it tells how to understand the signs of illness or injury your cat may develop and how to evaluate those signs in order to begin proper treatment. It resembles *The Well Dog Book* (some sections are exactly the same, where they apply equally to dogs and cats) since the two books were planned as companion volumes. Both are intended to help you understand what your veterinarian is talking about when they discuss your pet's health, to enable you to treat some illnesses at home, to prevent others, and truly to help your pet get well when an illness is too severe to be treated without professional skills. So this book is a kind of paramedic's handbook which should help you save money wasted in unnecessary veterinary visits, without endangering your pet's health.

For the most part I've covered only common health problems affecting cats here. I've tried to answer those questions cat owners most often ask me about cat care. I've tried not to oversimplify things, but in many cases technical information I thought the average cat owner would not be interested in or would not be likely to use is not included. If you are interested in details on certain subjects, go to some of the references mentioned in the text or ask your veterinarian for titles of other books that might help you. Use the information in this book to learn how to use your veterinarian as a resource. Remember, however, the book is not intended as a substitute for visits to the veterinarian, but rather as a supplement to them. Show this book to your

2

veterinarian as a sign that you are interested in taking an active part in maintaining your cat's health.

You don't need to buy any specialized equipment to use this book. Your eyes, hands, ears, and nose, and an understanding relationship with your cat are your most important tools. Don't be afraid to use them. There are more similarities between cats and people than many pet owners realize. As you read, you will probably find out that you know a lot more about "cat medicine" than you think you do.

The best way to use this book is to read it through at least once from beginning to end. In this way you will learn what is normal for your cat and how to take care of them when healthy, then the things that can indicate illness and what you should do about them. With this first reading you will find out which sections of the book you would like to read again and which sections you will only need to refer to if a specific problem arises. When you want to use this book to learn about a specific problem your cat may have, look for the problem in the General Index (page 263) and in the Index of Signs (page 113). To learn how to use these indices see page 107.

Anatomy is the place to begin. With this section as a guide you will learn a ready familiarity with your cat's body, and how to give them a physical exam. You may wish to refer back to this section when diagnosing an illness as well.

Preventive Medicine is a general health care section covering important aspects of your cat's daily life. It and the following sections have been designed for easy frequent reference by the use of running titles in the margins.

Diagnostic Medicine is the heart of the book. Be sure to read enough of this section to understand how it is organized and how to use the Index of Signs that precedes it. Then, when your cat shows any sign of illness or injury, use this section as a guide to proper action.

Home Medical Care tells you the basics of home treatment. It includes general nursing procedures and advice on drugs. Since in most cases of illness or injury your cat will have some treatment at home, you may want to become familiar with the information here before beginning to diagnose signs.

Breeding and Reproduction contains facts about the cat's reproductive cycle. Use it to learn how to prevent or plan pregnancy, how to care for a female before, during and after birth, and how to care for newborn or orphan kittens.

You, Your Cat and Your Veterinarian will help you if you don't yet have a veterinarian or are dissatisfied with your present one. Use it to learn what I think are characteristics of good veterinarians and what I think most veterinarians like to see in their clients.

The body always tries to heal itself. This important fact will help your treatment when your cat is sick. In many cases your cat will not need veterinary aid. Remember though, that by electing to treat your cat at home, you are taking responsibility for the results. Learn to recognize when the body is losing the battle to heal itself. If you can't be *sure* you are really helping your cat, discuss the problem with a doctor of veterinary medicine. Another caution: medicine is not always black or white. Usually there are several equally good ways to approach most health problems. I've recommended the approach that works for me; your veterinarian may disagree and get equal success with other methods. Trust your veterinarian and your common sense.

In several places throughout this book you will come across what seem to be unusual uses of the pronouns they, their *and* them. *These words have been chosen to avoid the use of gendered pronouns when referring to an indefinite person. Any inconvenience caused by this practice was felt to be outweighed by the benefits to be gained from it.*

4

Anatomy —
Getting to Know Your Cat's Body

Muscle and Bone
Skin
Eyes
Ears
Digestive System
Reproductive and Urinary Organs
Respiratory System
Heart and Blood
Nervous and Endocrine Systems

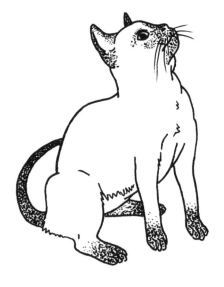

Anatomy

You can do a better job of giving your cat health care at home with some basic knowledge of *anatomy* and *physiology*. *Anatomy* is the structure of your cat's body and the relationships between its parts. For example, knowing the location of your cat's eyes and ears and their normal appearance is knowing anatomy. *Physiology* is the knowledge of how the parts of your cat's body function. Understanding how your cat's eyes and ears function to enable your cat to see and hear is an example of understanding physiology. Although you will be able to examine and understand anatomy easily, physiology is much more difficult. Brief descriptions of how your cat's various body parts work are given here, but it takes intensive study, such as that your veterinarian has given the subject, to really understand physiology well.

You will be most concerned with the external anatomy of your cat, but I've included some internal anatomy as well since an introduction to it will help you understand your veterinarian more easily as you discuss health problems your cat may have. The easiest and fastest way for you to become familiar with what you need to know is to get together with your cat and the following pages of this book. Handle your cat as you read the anatomical descriptions and look at the drawings. If you have a kitten, examine them several times as they grow. You will see many changes over several months and the physical contact will bring you closer to one another.

Looking carefully at your cat's anatomy and encouraging your cat to sit quietly while you examine them are extremely important in preparing both yourself and your cat for times when you will have to give health care at home. Also, the maneuvers you go through in examining your cat at home are the same ones your veterinarian uses when they give your cat a physical examination. A cat who has become accustomed to such handling at home is usually more relaxed and cooperative at the veterinary office.

For examination, place your cat on a smooth-surfaced table in good light. The smooth surface prevents good traction and, therefore, a "quick get away," and the novelty (at least for some cats) of being on a table will entice them to stay put rather than attempt an escape. Use a gentle touch and a minimum of restraint. Most cats respond poorly to heavy restraint: a hand placed gently over or in front of the shoulders or under the chest is usually sufficient. If your cat squirms and tries to get away, interrupt the exam, lift them quickly off their feet while voicing the command "No!" firmly, then replace them on the table. Don't give up. Although cats don't seem to be as naturally inclined to respond to obedience training as dogs, they can and do learn to respond to your wishes if you make them known clearly and are consistent. Be sure to praise your cat whenever they cooperate and repeat the correction procedure whenever they try to escape. The best procedure for a very uncooperative cat is to start out with very short exam periods, repeated frequently. As the cat becomes accustomed to the procedure and reassured that no injury is going to occur, they will become more cooperative and the examination time can be increased. There are several methods of firm restraint for use with cats (see page 203), but I think these should be reserved for use in the veterinarian's office or when you have to administer "disagreeable" treatment to your cat. Rely on consistent repetition and gentle handling to establish a good working relationship with your cat.

Physical Examination

Physical examination consists of applying knowledge of anatomy in a routine and thorough inspection of all or part of your cat's body. Each person (including every veterinarian) develops their own method for giving a physical examination. The best routine to develop is one which prevents you from forgetting to examine any part and one with which you feel most comfortable.

> Example: Examine your cat by systems as set out in *Anatomy* (muscle and bone, digestive system, etc.) Then return to examine miscellaneous items such as eyes, ears, and lymph nodes. Then take the cat's temperature.

> Example: Take the cat's temperature. Proceed with examination starting with the head and working towards the tail. In addition to examining special structures in the area, e.g., ears, eyes, mouth and nose for the head, toenails and pads for the limbs, don't forget to examine the skin in each area and to look for the lymph nodes associated with each area. Follow up by watching your cat in motion.

Special tools needed for physical examination: A rectal thermometer is the only special tool necessary for performing a routine physical examination of your cat at home. Your other tools are your five senses, particularly the senses of touch, sight, and smell.

Special terms used in physical examination: Except for anatomical names of body parts which are mentioned and illustrated in *Anatomy*, there are few special terms that you need to learn to help you with a physical examination. Refer to this page if any of the following words are confusing in the text:

> *palpate* — to examine with your hands. This is one of

your most important methods of physical examination and is why you are asked to *palpate* or *feel* parts of your cat's body so frequently throughout this book.

Terms which indicate direction in reference to the body are illustrated below.

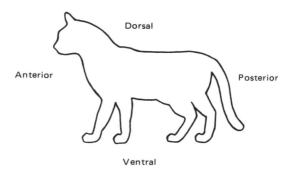

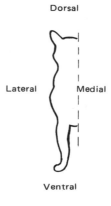

Muscle and Bone
(The *Musculoskeletal* System)

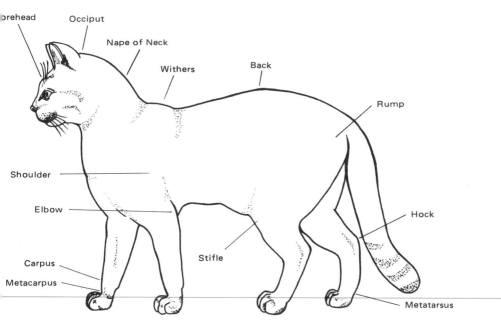

Muscle tissue is composed of contractile units which provide the power for voluntary movement, breathing, blood circulation, digestion, glandular secretion, excretion of body wastes and many other more minor functions as well. There are three types of muscle tissue in your cat's body. *Smooth* or *unstriated* muscle is involved in a host of primarily involuntary body functions such as the *peristaltic* (wave-like) movements of the digestive tract. *Cardiac* (heart) muscle, which is capable of independent rhythmic contraction, is found only in the heart, the pump of the circulatory system. *Skeletal* or *striated* muscle makes up the rest of the muscles in the body. including the diaphragm and certain trunk muscles responsible for breathing. An illustration of the muscles in your cat's body is not included in this book because knowing their positions and names is not important in giving routine health care at home.

11

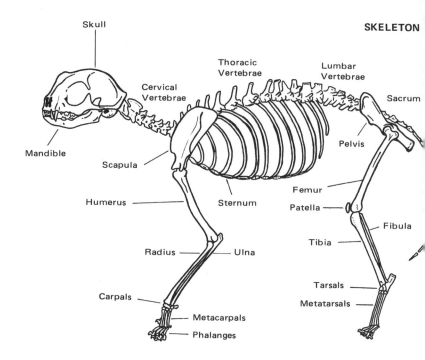

Skull

Thoracic Vertebrae

Cervical Vertebrae

Lumbar Vertebrae

Sacrum

Mandible

Scapula

Pelvis

Humerus

Sternum

Femur

Patella

Fibula

Radius

Ulna

Tibia

Carpals

Tarsals

Metatarsals

Metacarpals

Phalanges

Bone is a continually changing and actively metabolizing tissue in the living animal. It is composed primarily of the minerals calcium and phosphorus in an organic connective tissue framework which is mainly protein. The outstanding physical functions of bone are 1) to form the skeleton which supports and protects the soft tissues (e.g., organs, muscles, fat) of the body, and 2) to provide levers against which the various skeletal muscles move. The bones have other functions as well: mineral storage is provided in the hard bone itself, and fat storage and the formation of blood cells occur in the marrow present inside the bones. Each cat has about 244 bones in their

CUT-AWAY VIEW OF LONG BONE

Cartilage

Marrow Cavity

Cortex

skeletal structure. Names of bones which might be important to you in understanding your veterinarian's diagnosis are marked on the skeletal drawing. See whether you can locate each of them on your cat with your hands.

Start with the *skull* (head); notice its compact, round shape and short, powerful jaws. Thick and thin layers of muscle and connective tissue overlie the bones of the skull, but these tissues are not very prominent and you may have difficulty distinguishing between the soft tissues and bone. You may be able to feel the relatively thick, paired *temporal* muscles over the top of the head between the ears, and the *masseter* muscles which lie in the area of your cat's cheeks. These two pairs of muscles function together with smaller muscles to close the mouth. The rest of the skull feels very bony. Trace the bony area between the temporal muscles back to its end behind the ears. This small, hard bump at the end is called the *occipital protuberance* and is a normal part of every cat's skull. Another bony area easy to identify is the *mandible*; it forms the lower jaw. You move this bone when opening and closing your cat's mouth (see page 28).

The skull is attached to the rest of the skeleton by the *cervical vertebrae*. Try to feel these neck bones by moving your fingers firmly over the sides and top of the neck. You will find it very difficult to feel any bony structures because of the well-developed muscles which cover the neck. The cervical vertebrae along with the lower vertebrae form your cat's *spinal column* (backbone).

The *thoracic vertebrae* start in the area between the edges of the shoulder blades. You can feel the curved upper edge of each *scapula* (shoulder blade) near the middle of the back at the *withers*. Each scapula and the muscles which cover it can be seen to move freely when your cat walks and runs. Use your index finger to feel the spines of the thoracic vertebrae between the shoulder blades. Unless your cat is pretty fat you will be able to trace these bones with your finger down the center of your cat's back. They become the spines of the *lumbar vertebrae* in the area behind the last rib and disappear near the hip where several vertebrae are joined to form the *sacrum*. You can feel only the spines of the

13

vertebral bones but not the rest of the bones themselves because a heavy group of muscles lies on each side of the spinal column down the back. These *epaxial* muscles are most prominent in the *lumbar* region where you can feel them easily by running your fingers along each side of the spinal column. Unless your cat is tailless, you will probably be able to feel each *coccygeal* (tail) vertebrae under its covering muscles.

Now examine each leg starting at the foot. The average cat has five *digits* (toes) on each of the front feet and four each on the back feet. Cats affected with *polydactyly,* an inherited trait, may have from one to four extra digits on the front feet, but extra toes on the rear feet are quite rare. Feel each toe carefully. You will find that each consists of three bones *(phalanges)*. These correspond to the bones in your fingers and toes. The first toe bone (first phalanx) and nail are covered by a fold of skin in the relaxed foot. These retractile nails allow your cat to walk quietly. To examine these, grasp the leg in the palm of your hand, place your index finger on the pad of the toe you want to examine and your thumb over the top of the same toe at the joint between the first and second phalanx, then squeeze your fingers together. When you do this you will find that the toenail and first phalanx come into view and will remain extended until you release your fingers. Move your fingers slowly up each toe to the middle of the foot. In this area each toe is attached to a long bone which corresponds to the bones that form the palm of your

EXTENDING THE CLAW

CLAW MECHANISM

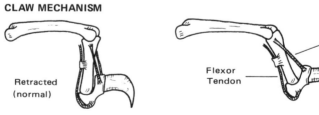

Retracted (normal)

Elastic Ligament

Flexor Tendon

Extended

hand and the sole of your foot. These bones are called *metacarpals* in the front feet and *metatarsals* in the rear.

14

The *forepaw* (front foot) attaches to the *foreleg* (front leg) at the *carpus* (wrist). Gently flex and extend this joint. If you *palpate* (examine with your hands) carefully, you may be able to feel the small individual bones which form this joint. Above the carpus are the long bones of the *forearm*, the *radius* and *ulna*. These bones are well covered by muscles on the *lateral* (outside) surfaces except in the region of the elbow, but if you feel deeply you will be able to feel bone through the muscle layers. On the *medial* (inside) surface you can easily feel bone (the radius) near the wrist. Place the fingers of one hand over the elbow. Grasp the forearm with your other hand and flex and extend the joint. A normal joint moves smoothly causing no grating or grinding vibrations to be felt in your fingers. The *humerus* is the bone which forms the foreleg above the elbow. It is well-covered with muscles that correspond to those in your upper arm. The humerus is most easy to feel at the point of the shoulder, but if you feel deeply in other areas you can also find it underlying the muscles.

REAR LEG

Femur

Patella

Gastrocnemius Muscle

Fibula

Tibia

Achille's Tendon

In the *hindlimb* (rear leg) the foot attaches to the leg at the *hock*. This joint corresponds to your ankle. Flex and extend the joint to learn its normal movement. The fibrous band which attaches prominently on the posterior surface of the hock is the "Achilles tendon." It is part of a mechanism which causes the hock to flex or extend whenever the *stifle* (knee) is flexed or extended and vice versa. The *tibia* and *fibula* are the bones which lie between the knee and the hock. Muscles cover the *lateral* (outside) surface of these bones, but you can feel them through the muscles and can easily feel the tibia on the inside surface of the leg in this area. The tibia helps to form the *stifle* (knee) joint along with the *femur* and *patella* (kneecap). Place the fingers of one hand over the patella and

15

flex and extend the knee joint. You should be able to feel the patella move freely and smoothly as you manipulate the joint. Now move up the leg to the thigh. The *femur* is the long bone of the thigh. It is well-covered by heavy muscles, so you will be unable to feel it easily except near the knee. Feel the muscles of the thigh and try to feel the femur under them. The femur *articulates* (forms a joint) with the pelvis at the hip. To test this joint, grasp the thigh with the fingers and palm of one hand and place your thumb over the area of the hip joint, then flex and extend the joint. This leaves one hand free to control your cat. You can perform this part of the examination either with your cat standing on three legs or lying on one side. Complete your examination of the musculoskeletal system by running your fingers over the sides of your cat's chest. You should be able to feel each rib easily under a freely moveable coat of skin, fat and muscle. If you can't easily feel the ribs, your cat is too fat. Pick a rib and follow it with your fingers down the side of the *thorax* (chest) to its end. If you have chosen one of the first nine ribs you will find that it attaches to a bone forming the *ventral* (bottom) surface of the chest. This is the *sternum*. The last four ribs do not attach directly to the sternum.

EXAMINATION
OF THE HIP JOINT

After you have examined the major parts of your cat's musculoskeletal system (or before if you like), stand back and look at your cat as a whole. Are the legs straight? Are the wrist joints erect? Are there any unusual lumps or bumps? Most normal cats are very similar in *conformation* (bony and muscular structure) to the drawings in this book.

Now watch your cat move. All motion should be free and effortless. Do you see any signs of lameness? If you have any particular questions about your cat's conformation or movement be sure to discuss them with your veterinarian.

16

Skin
(The *Integumentary* System)

The integumentary system consists of the skin and its specialized modifications: the hair, the footpads, the claws and the anal sacs. Your cat's skin protects their body against environmental changes, trauma and germs. In the skin vitamin D is synthesized; below the skin (in the *subcutaneous* tissues) fat is stored. Skin is both an organ of sensation and an organ (via certain skin glands) for waste excretion. Unlike humans' skin however, the cat's body skin plays only a minor role in heat regulation. Skin disease does occur in cats, and the condition of your cat's skin and hair can sometimes tell you a great deal about their body's general state of health.

If your cat is healthy, their skin should be smooth, pliable and free from large amounts of scales (dandruff), scabs, odorous secretions and parasites (see page 95). Normal skin coloration ranges from pale pink through shades of brown to black. Spotted skin is completely normal and may be seen in cats without spotted coats. The skin (and hair) color comes from a dark-colored pigment called *melanin* which is produced and stored in special cells in the bottom layer of the *epidermis* (outer skin layer).

Examine your cat's skin carefully. To do this, part the fur of long-haired cats in several places and look carefully at the skin itself. In short-haired cats run the thumb of one hand against the grain of the hair to expose the skin. Be sure to examine the skin in several places over the body, on the legs, under the neck and on the head. When you are examining the head, note how there is a distinct thinning of hair in front of the ears. This is called *preauricular alopecia;* although the degree varies between cats, its presence is normal. It marks the site of the temporal glands, microscopic skin glands thought to be important in scent marking. Any bug-like

PREAURICULAR ALOPECIA

Sparse Hair Cover

17

creatures you see attached to your cat's skin or hair or which quickly move away as you part the hair are *external parasites* and should not be there. They are likely to be fleas (see page 95), but may be lice (see page 99), mites (see page 99) or ticks (see page 98). Small salt and pepper-like, black and white granules present may be flea eggs and flea feces.

A specialized area of skin of particular interest to owners of mature tomcats is the *supracaudal organ*. This is an area of numerous and large oil producing glands located on the upper surface of the tail. Although it is present in all cats, it is not particularly evident unless there is excessive accumulation of the gland's oily secretion. If this has occurred in your cat, you will find an area of greasy, brownish secretion as you part the hair on the top of the tail. This may be accompanied by stringy, oily hairs. This unsightly condition is referred to as *stud tail* and is sometimes relieved by castration (see page 225).

SUPRACAUDAL GLAND

Roll your cat on their side or back to see where the skin forms the nipples of the *mammary glands* (breasts). The mammary glands themselves are skin glands which have become modified for the production of milk. Male as well as female cats normally have four nipples on each side, although some cats have as many as five pairs. The prominence of the nipples and mammary glands in the *queen* (female cat) varies with age and stage of the *estrous cycle* (see page 219). Examine your cat's mammary glands by feeling the areas between the nipples and a wide area around them. In a normal male or *anestrous female* (see page 219) you should not be able to feel any lumps or bumps. If you find *any*, discuss their importance with your veterinarian.

If you have a young cat with short abdominal hair, you may notice a faint scar-like area on the skin at the midline near the area where the chest meets the *abdomen* (belly) while you are examining the breasts. This is your cat's *umbilicus* (belly button). If you see a lump in this area, it

18

may be an *umbilical hernia* (see page 246 and decide whether or not you need a veterinarian's help).

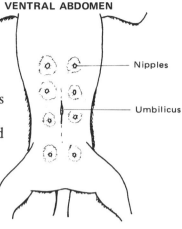

Nipples

Umbilicus

Now return to the head to examine your cat's nose. The skin is modified over the nose so that its superficial layers are thick and tough. This skin has no glands, but is usually moist from nasal secretions and feels cool as a result of evaporation. A cool moist nose or a warm dry one, however, is not an accurate gauge of your cat's body temperature; use a thermometer! (See page 194.) Cats' noses vary widely in coloration. Colors anywhere from salmon or pale pink through brown to black are normal, as are spotted noses. A brightly colored nose which becomes pale or white can be a sign of illness (see page 163) so be sure to become familiar with the normal appearance of your cat's nose.

The skin is also modified to be thick and tough over the footpads. The deepest layer of the footpads is very fatty and acts as a cushion to absorb shock. The middle layer (*dermis*) contains *eccrine glands*: the only skin glands in the cat equivalent to humans' heat-regulating sweat glands. If you feel your cat's footpads when they become excited (e.g., on a trip to the veterinarian's office) you will find that the pads become damp with eccrine gland secretion. These glands are also responsible for the steamy footprints you may see when your cat crosses the sidewalk on a warm day.

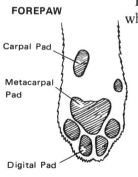

FOREPAW

Carpal Pad

Metacarpal Pad

Digital Pad

The footpads are named according to which bones they overlie—*digital, metacarpal* (*metatarsal* in the rear feet) and *carpal* (none in the rear). Examine your cat's footpads and learn the names. Knowing the names may help you describe the location of a problem to your veterinarian.

Two unusual modifications

19

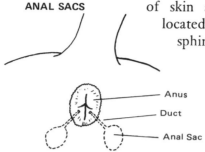

ANAL SACS

Anus

Duct

Anal Sac

of skin are the *anal sacs.* They are located internally under the external sphincter muscles of the anus at about four o'clock and eight o'clock. If you lift your cat's tail directly upward you can see the small opening where each duct empties on each side near the opening of the anus. If the glands are full, a drop of two of brownish fluid will often drip from the openings as you lift the tail. This odorous anal sac secretion may serve to mark your cat's stool with their particular identification tag. You may be able to feel the full anal sacs by placing your thumb externally on one side of the anus and your index finger on the other side, then gently moving your fingers up and down. Full glands feel like firm, dried pea-sized objects beneath the skin. Rarely a cat's anal sacs don't empty properly on their own: then you or your veterinarian must empty them (see page 153).

Claws (toenails) are specialized in cats for digging, traction and protection. To examine your cat's claws, extend them as explained on page 14.

CROSS SECTION OF CLAW

Claw   Ungual Process
        Dermis (Quick)

3rd Phalanx

2nd Phalanx

Pad

The outer layer of the claw is horny and may be pigmented or unpigmented. The inner layer is the *dermis* (quick) which is highly *vascular* (contains mainly blood vessels) and continuous with the connective tissue covering the third phalanx. Even in a dark-nailed cat you can usually see the dermis as a pink area inside the claw when it is held in front of a light. Cats normally keep their claws sharp by constant conditioning through which the old, dulled and worn outer layers of the claws are pulled off. This normal scratching behavior sometimes becomes undesirable in cats

20

confined indoors. Providing a cat with their own scratching post, nail trimming or declawing (see page 56) are ways to help solve the problem.

Cats have three basic types of hair: guard hair, fine hair and tactile hair. *Tactile hairs* (whiskers) grow out of very large sensory hair follicles on the muzzle and chin, at the sides of the face, and over the eyes. Their sensory function is a significant aid to your cat's vision and hearing and is thought to be of particular importance in helping a cat orient themselves in poor light. *Guard hairs* are the longer, coarser hairs which comprise the outer part of your cat's coat. *Fine hairs* are the soft hairs which make up the undercoat. Unless your cat is a *Rex*, a special breed with a coat composed only of fine, curly hairs, whether the coat is long or short there are both guard hairs and fine hairs present. Try to distinguish between them in your cat's coat.

Although you may notice a particular increase in the numbers of hairs your cats sheds in the spring, all cats' coats are replacing themselves continuously. At any one time some hairs are falling out, some are in a resting phase, and others are growing in. Don't consider shedding excessive unless you begin to see bare skin areas developing in normally-haired sites. A healthy cat's coat is neatly groomed and clean (although tomcats often look very dirty and unkempt when healthy). The coat should appear glossy and unbroken. Dark-colored coats usually seem to have more natural sheen, so take this into consideration before judging your cat's coat. After clipping or shaving, the average cat's coat takes three to four months to regrow, but it can take much longer especially in long-haired cats.

Eyes

Your cat's eyes are similar in structure and function to your own. Light entering the eye passes through the cornea, anterior chamber, pupil, lens and vitreous body before striking the retina. Specialized cells in the retina (the rods and cones) convert light striking them into nervous signals

EYEBALL

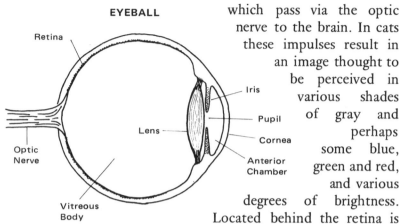

Retina

Optic Nerve

Lens

Iris

Pupil

Cornea

Anterior Chamber

Vitreous Body

which pass via the optic nerve to the brain. In cats these impulses result in an image thought to be perceived in various shades of gray and perhaps some blue, green and red, and various degrees of brightness. Located behind the retina is an area of tissue called the *tapetum lucidum*. Its function is to reflect light which has already passed through the rods and cones back to them again (increasing visual acuity in dim light). It is the structure which is responsible for the appearance of cats' eyes "glowing in the dark."

As you examine your cat's eyes you will see that each is surrounded by two modified skin folds, the eyelids. The edges of the lids should be smooth, even and not rolled in (*entropion*) or out (*ectropion*). Cats do

Normal Eye Lids   Entropion   Ectropion

not normally have eyelashes. Look for lashes on your cat's eyelids and if any are present, be sure that they do not turn in abnormally to rub against the eye. Between the eyelids at the *medial canthus* (corner of the eye near the nose) you can see the third eyelid (*nictitating membrane*). It may be pale pink or partially pigmented. Its normal position over the eye

EXTERNAL EYE

Medial Canthus

3rd Eyelid

Iris

Lateral Canthus

Sclera

Pupil

varies from cat to cat and has some relationship to the presence of disease (see page 131). Roll back the upper or lower eyelid by placing your thumb near its edge and gently pulling upward or downward. This allows you to view the inner lining of the lids, a pale pink mucuous membrane called the *conjunctiva.*

EXAMINING THE EYE

Swollen 3rd Eyelid

Inflamed Sclera

Conjunctiva (forms conjunctival sac when lid released)

The visible part of the eyeball consists of the cornea, bulbar conjunctiva, anterior chamber, iris and pupil. The *bulbar conjunctiva* is a continuation of the lining of the eyelids. If it contains pigment the area may look spotted or dark. In unpigmented areas the bulbar conjunctiva is transparent, allowing the eye's white fibrous coat *(sclera)* and

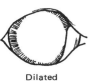

Dilated Pupil

Constricted Pupil

the fine blood vessels which traverse it to be seen through it. The cornea should be completely transparent. Through it you see the anterior chamber, iris and pupil. The color of the iris varies widely among cats. Greens and yellows predominate, but many other iris colors are possible, among them orange, blue, and lavender. The iris controls the size and shape of the pupil. Along with the eyelids, the pupil controls the amount of light allowed to enter the eye. Pupils should constrict simultaneously in bright light and dilate in dim light. When only one eye is exposed to light or darkness, the pupil of the remaining eye should constrict or dilate when the exposed one does. If your cat's eyes are normal, you will find that the pupils are round when dilated, slit-like (vertically) when constricted when you test their response to light.

23

Ears

The external part of the ear, which you can see when casually looking at your cat, is called the *pinna*. The pinna receives air vibrations and transmits them via the ear canal to the eardrum. The outside of the pinna is covered with haired skin like that covering the rest of your cat's body. The inside is also partially haired, although the hair there is more sparse than that on the outside. Any visible unpigmented skin lining the inside of the pinna and ear canal should be pale pink in color. Bright pink or red is abnormal. All visible parts of the ear should be fairly clean. Normal accumulations consist of a small amount of yellowish to brown waxy material. Large amounts of this material, black waxy material, or sticky foul-smelling secretions are abnormal. If your cat's ears look normal to you, or your veterinarian tells you that your cat's ears are normal, smell them. This odor is the smell of a healthy ear. Deviations from this smell may indicate ear trouble even if you can't see any external indication of it.

Notice on the drawing that the ear canal is vertical for a distance, then becomes horizontal before it reaches the

24

eardrum. This makes it impossible for you or your veterinarian to see very deeply into the ear canal without a special instrument called an *otoscope.* An advantage of this type of ear canal structure is that it allows you to clean quite deeply into the ear canal without fear of damaging the eardrum as long as you clean vertically (see page 202).

The structure and function of your cat's middle and inner ear are very similar to your own. Vibrations reaching the eardrum are transmitted through the middle ear by small bones, the *auditory ossicles,* to the oval window. From the oval window the vibrations enter the inner ear where the cochlea converts these mechanical stimuli to nervous impulses which travel to the brain via the auditory nerve. In addition to the cochlea, the semicircular canals and utricle occupy the inner ear. These organs are important in maintaining the cat's sense of balance.

The Digestive System
(The *Gastrointestinal* Tract)

The digestive system consists of the digestive tube (mouth, pharynx, esophagus, stomach, small and large intestines, and anus) and the associated salivary glands, liver and gall bladder and pancreas. Few of the foodstuffs necessary for growth, life and work enter the body in a form that can be absorbed directly by the intestines and put straight to use by the body. Therefore it is the digestive system's function to convert foodstuffs to absorbable nutrients, using both mechanical and chemical means.

Anatomically you will be

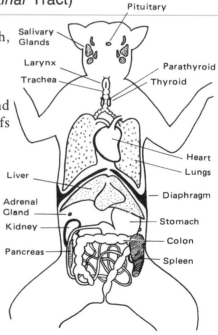

OCTOSCOPE

Pituitary

Salivary Glands

Larynx

Trachea

Parathyroid

Thyroid

Heart

Lungs

Liver

Diaphragm

Adrenal Gland

Kidney

Stomach

Colon

Pancreas

Spleen

25

primarily concerned with the beginning and end of the digestive tract—the mouth and anus. The locations of the other structures are indicated on the drawing of internal anatomy. With practice you may become quite familiar with the shape and feel of some of the internal organs because most cats are small enough and have relaxed enough abdomens to make palpation easy. Feel *gently* and carefully; too firm or rough an examination can cause injury to your cat. With your cat standing, feel for the liver and stomach by running your fingers down the edges of the ribs bordering the

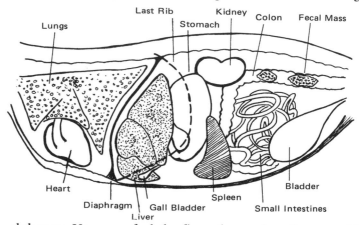

abdomen. You may feel the firm, sharp edge of a normal liver most easily along the rib edge on the right side. Round liver edges or a liver which extends for some distance beyond the rib may be abnormal. When full, your cat's stomach will be felt as a doughy or lumpy mass against the left side of the abdomen near the rib. You will also encounter the spleen (see page 38 on the left side. Feel your cat's intestines by grasping the abdomen between the thumb and fingers of one hand. Reach up along each side of the abdomen, bring your thumb and fingers towards one another, then move them downward. The intestines will slip through your fingers like wet noodles. If you reach high up in the posterior (towards the tail) part of the abdomen you may be able to feel your cat's colon full of stool. It will feel firm and somewhat sausage-shaped. If you become familiar with the shape and feel of a normal stool in your cat's colon, it may help you in

26

the diagnosis of diarrhea (see page 150) or constipation (see page 151). As you perform your examination of the digestive system, you are likely to encounter the kidneys and bladder. For information about these organs turn to page 31.

Mouth

Most cats are reluctant to have their mouths examined, especially the first time. Don't give up if your cat objects and tries to squirm away as you start your examination. Make your intentions clear and proceed with an air of confidence. If you are hesitant in your motions most cats will be quick to take advantage of the situation. Begin the examination by lifting each upper lip individually with the jaws closed. Use one hand to steady your cat's head, if necessary, while examining with the other. This allows you to examine the *buccal* (outer) surfaces of the teeth and gums.

Healthy gums feel firm and have edges so closely applied to the teeth that they look as if they are actually attached to the teeth. They fill the upper part of the spaces between teeth, form- ing a "V" (an inverted "V" with

Healthy Gums   Severe Gum Disease

the lower teeth) which you can see between each front tooth and its neighbors. In unpigmented areas healthy gums are pink. Very pale pink or white gums, yellowish gums, red gums, or a red line along the tooth edge of pink gums is abnormal. Many normal cats have black spotted gums, some with so much pigment that it is difficult to find a pink area to examine.

Cats' teeth are designed for grasping, tearing and shredding. In a normal mouth, the upper front teeth (incisors) just overlap the lower ones. An excessive overlap (overbite) is abnormal, as is a mouth structure in which the lower front teeth extend beyond the upper ones (underbite). A mild overbite or underbite doesn't seem to cause func- tional problems. Be sure to check your cat's bite and the surface of each tooth. The surfaces of the teeth are white in young cats and get yellower as the cat ages. A fingernail scraped along tooth surfaces should pick up little debris. Try it. Mushy white stuff that may scrape off is called *plaque* or *materia alba.* This can be removed easily by "brushing" your cat's teeth (see page 57). Hard white, yellow or brown material is *tartar* or *calculus* and must usually be removed by your veterinarian.

Teeth are catagorized into four types: incisors (I), canines (C), premolars (P) and molars (M). Veterinarians use a formula to indicate the number and placement of each kind of tooth in the mouth. A letter indicates the kind of tooth; the numbers placed next to the letter indicate how many of that particular kind of tooth are present in the upper and lower jaw of one-half of the mouth. The average kitten has twenty-six *deciduous* teeth (baby teeth) arranged in the following manner: Starting at the middle of the front teeth (incisors)

Canine

Incisors

Premolars   Molar

$$\frac{\text{Upper teeth of } \frac{1}{2} \text{ mouth}}{\text{Lower teeth of } \frac{1}{2} \text{ mouth}} = I\frac{3}{3}, \ C\frac{1}{1}, \ P\frac{3}{2}.$$

A kitten has no molars. Therefore the eruption of these baby teeth and their replacement by permanent ones is a convenient way to estimate the age of a young cat (see table page 29).

The average adult cat has thirty permanent teeth:

$$\frac{\text{Upper teeth of } \frac{1}{2} \text{ mouth}}{\text{Lower teeth of } \frac{1}{2} \text{ mouth}} = I\frac{3}{3}, \ C\frac{1}{1}, \ P\frac{3}{2}, \ M\frac{1}{1}.$$

It is not unusual to find cats with fewer teeth than this "standard" number. Many cats never develop the full number of incisor teeth, others lose these teeth relatively early in life. If the other teeth and the gums are healthy, this doesn't seem to cause any problems. Once a cat's permanent teeth have erupted it is more difficult to use them as a guide to age.

OPENING THE MOUTH

Now examine the inner *(lingual)* surfaces of the teeth, the tongue and the posterior part of the mouth. *To open your cat's mouth,* place one hand around the upper part of their head and push inward on the upper lips with your fingers and thumb as if you were trying to push them between the teeth. As your cat starts to open their mouth, use the index finger of your other hand to pull open the lower jaw by pushing downward on the lower incisor teeth. Look inside. You will see the rough surface of the tongue below, the hard palate above, and the inner teeth surfaces. If you move quickly you can use your finger to push the tongue to one side or the other to look under it. Using the index finger of the same hand you used to open the lower jaw, press down on the tongue. As you press down, try to move the tongue slightly forward. If you do this properly, you will mimic your doctor's use of a tongue depressor, allowing you to see the soft palate as a continuation of the hard palate, and the palantine tonsils. Cats' tonsils reside in a pocket (the *tonsilar crypt* or *sinus*), so they aren't easily seen unless they are enlarged.

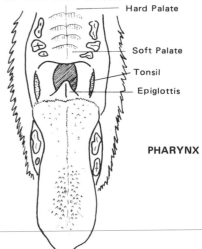

Hard Palate

Soft Palate

Tonsil

Epiglottis

PHARYNX

Teeth As a Guide To Your Cat's Age

Age	Teeth Present
Birth	None
2-3 weeks	Deciduous teeth coming in
4-5 weeks	All deciduous teeth in
3½-4½ months	Permanent incisors coming in
5 months	Permanent canines erupt
6 months	Premolar 3 present

Rarely, deciduous teeth may be retained as the permanent ones erupt. These may have to be removed by a veterinarian if they interfere with normal adult tooth placement.

After one year of age some staining and tartar accumulations are usually present on the teeth. There is no reliable way to use teeth as a guide to age, however, after a cat is mature.

Tonsils are a type of specialized *lymphoid* tissue (containing many special cells called lymphocytes, see page 76) similar to your lymph nodes and to lymph nodes located in other parts of your cat's body. You can feel some lymph nodes on your cat's head in the area located below your cat's ear and behind the cheek where the head attaches to the neck. They are very small, firm, smooth-surfaced lumps associated with a larger similar lump. The larger lump is one of the cat's several salivary glands, and the only one you will be able to feel. After you feel the normal salivary gland and its associated lymph nodes and become familiar with them, try to feel the other lymph nodes indicated on the drawing. (You may need your veterinarian's help with this; unless the nodes are enlarged they can be difficult to find the first time you try to feel them.) When you find one, learn its normal size and shape. Lymph node changes (most commonly enlargement) should alert you to have your cat examined by a veterinarian since they are often a sign of serious illness or infection.

Anus　　Just about everyone knows that the anus is the specialized terminal portion of the digestive tract through which indigestible material and waste products pass as stool. But some people have questions regarding what constitutes a normal bowel movement. Others are unaware of the anal sacs located in this area.

Most adult cats have one or two bowel movements daily. The number of bowel movements and the volume of stool passed, however, are dependent to a great degree on the amount of undigestible material in the diet. Cats eating dry food will tend to pass more feces than cats eating a highly digestible muscle meat, egg and milk product diet, due to the higher fiber content of dry cat food. Normal stools are well-formed and generally colored brown, although some diet ingredients may make them darker (liver) or lighter (bones). Extremely large volumes of stool, unformed, abnormally

30

odorous stools, or unusually colored stools may indicate digestive tract disease. Be sure to try to observe your cat's stools several times a week.

Anal sacs have been discussed with the skin: see page 20. If you have not yet examined them, do it now while learning the normal appearance of your cat's anus. You may also want to learn to take your cat's temperature at this time since it should be a routine part of any physical examination and must be taken rectally (see page 194).

Reproductive and Urinary Organs
(The *Genitourinary* System)

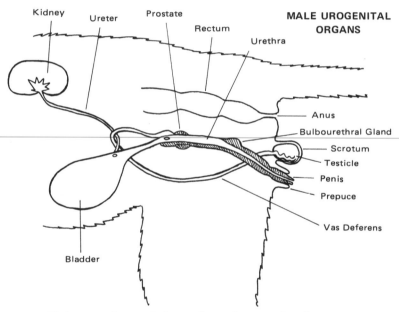

Kidney Ureter Prostate Rectum Urethra **MALE UROGENITAL ORGANS**

Anus
Bulbourethral Gland
Scrotum
Testicle
Penis
Prepuce
Vas Deferens
Bladder

Major portions of the male cat's reproductive system are located externally within reach of your examination. Many cats resist a thorough examination of their genitals, however, so don't feel dismayed if you can't examine all parts as described. The *testes* (organs which produce sperm) are located in the *scrotum* of the male (skin pouch containing the testes) at birth and should be relatively easy to feel by six weeks of age. Normally there are two testicles present, each

31

of which feels firm, smooth and relatively oval beneath its loose covering of skin. If your cat has one or no testicles in his scrotum *(monorchid* or *cryptorchid)* the condition may need veterinary attention (see page 227). If you palpate carefully, you can feel a small lump protruding off the posterior end of each testicle. This is the tail of the *epididymis* which stores sperm.

EXTRUDING THE PENIS

To examine your cat's penis you must first retract the skin fold which covers it (the *prepuce* or *sheath*). To do this, grasp the prepuce gently but firmly between the index finger and thumb of one hand. Then push the skin fold anteriorly toward your cat's head. As you do this you will see the pink tip of the penis start to protrude posteriorly; a cat's penis points toward the tail. If you have gotten a successful grip the first time, the rest of the penis will protrude once the skin fold is pushed fully forward and it will remain protruded as long as you hold the retracted skin in place. If you have difficulty retracting the sheath the first time, try getting a better grasp. Try several positions before giving up.

The surface of the penis is covered by a pink mucous membrane. Prominent curved, horny *papillae* protrude from its surface in the area of the *glans* (expanded end of the penis) in mature, uncastrated males (tomcats). It is thought that these rough projections may be involved in stimulating the female cat to ovulate following mating; they may also provide additional sexual stimulation to the male and act as a holdfast. If your cat is very young or castrated, you will find that the surface of the glans penis is smooth. The spines begin to develop at about two months of age and have usually disappeared by six months following castration. The *urethra* (tube through which urine and reproductive secretions pass) can be seen to open at the end of the penis. It is extremely

32

narrow in all male cats. If you see your cat urinate, notice what a thin stream of urine this produces. Any secretions present on the surface of the penis should be clear not cloudy or colored.

Sperm are produced in the seminiferous tubules of the testicles. From the testes the sperm travel to the epididymis for storage and maturation. During ejaculation sperm travel through the *vas deferens* into the urethra where they are mixed with secretions from the prostate gland and bulbourethral glands before exiting the penis. The prostate and bulbourethral glands are located internally and are not accessible for routine examination.

The vulva and clitoris are the only female cat's genitals which can be seen externally. The internal portions of the female reproductive tract—*uterus, cervix, ovaries* and *fallopian tubes*—can be found on the illustrations here. The urethra empties into the vagina anterior to a point you can see without special instruments. You may be able to see the tiny, dark pink clitoris in its fossa by gently spreading the

FEMALE REPRODUCTIVE SYSTEM

Ovary
Oviduct
Uterine Horn
Body of Uterus
Cervix
Vagina
Clitoris

VULVA

Vaginal Opening
Clitoris

FEMALE GENITAL ANATOMY

Colon
Ovary
Oviduct
Anus
Ureter
Vagina
Clitoris
Uterine Horn
Vulva
Cervix
Urethra
Bladder

vulvar lips with your fingers. This also allows you to see some of the lining of the vulva and vagina. These mucous membranes should be pink in color; any secretions present are normally clear.

You can find additional information on reproduction in the chapter *Breeding and Reproduction* starting on page 217.

The urinary system of both male and female cats consists of two kidneys, two ureters, the bladder and the urethra. Look for these organs on the illustrations. *Nephrons* (units of specialized cells) in the kidneys filter the blood to remove toxic metabolic wastes and are also important in maintaining the body's proper electrolyte and water balance. Urine formed in the kidneys passes through the ureters to the bladder where it is stored until it is eliminated through the urethra during urination. Normal cat urine is yellow and clear and has a distinctive odor. This odor is extremely intense in tomcats and is used to mark territory during the act of spraying (see page 161). The intensity of the yellow color of urine increases as the amount of water excreted decreases and vice versa. If your cat is not fat you will probably be able to feel their bladder and kidneys. With your cat standing, restrain them with one hand under the chest while using the other one to feel for the bladder in the posterior abdomen between the rear legs. A bladder containing urine will feel somewhat like a water-filled balloon varying anywhere from about the size of a Concord grape to the size of a lemon. Feel *gently* for the kidneys by grasping the abdomen with both hands, left on the left side, right hand on the right side. Reach high into the mid-lumbar area then bring your fingers towards one another. Each kidney should feel firm, smooth and relatively oval in shape. Most normal adult cat's kidneys are about the size of a small apricot, but there is much individual variation with body size. You may find the right kidney somewhat more anterior than the left one, but both move rather freely and will not be found in the exact same position with each examination.

Respiratory System

The cat's respiratory system consists of two lungs, the air passages leading to them (nasal cavity, mouth, pharynx, larynx, trachea, bronchi), the diaphragm and the muscles of the thorax. The system's main function, as in humans, is to supply oxygen to the body and to remove excess carbon dioxide produced by metabolism. In conjunction with the tongue and the mucous membranes of the mouth, the respiratory system has a secondary but extremely important function of heat regulation, since the cat has no highly developed mechanism for sweating.

The only parts of your cat's respiratory system you can see are the mouth and nostrils. Special instruments are needed to look into the nasal cavity and this is difficult, even with special instruments, because the passages are so small. Look at your cat's nostrils. Any secretions from them should be clear and watery; sticky, cloudy, yellowish or greenish nasal discharge is abnormal.

You can feel your cat's *larynx* (Adam's apple) by grasping their neck on the undersurface where it meets the head. The larynx feels like a small hard, fairly inflexible mass. It helps control the flow of air through the trachea and lungs and is the location of the vocal cords responsible for your cat's meow. It is thought that the cat's purr does not arise in this region, but is transmitted through the air passages after arising from vibratory motions occurring in the wall of a major blood vessel in the chest when the velocity and turbulence of blood flow is increased.

Notice the character of your cat's respirations at rest and after exercise. A normal cat at rest breathes about twenty to thirty times per minute. The movements of the chest are smooth and unstrained. After exercise, of course, the rate is much faster and on warm days or during periods of extreme excitement panting may occur. Changes in the rate and character of a cat's respiration may indicate disease. Be sure to become familiar with your cat's normal breathing at rest, on cool and warm days, during and after exercise so you can tell when changes from the normal have occurred.

Heart and Blood
(The *Circulatory* System)

Your cat's circulatory system is similar to your own. It consists of a four-chambered heart which serves as a blood pump, arteries which carry blood away from the heart to the capillaries where molecular exchange occurs, and veins which return blood to the heart. There are no direct methods you c an use to examine this system. A stethoscope (available at medical supply houses) will aid you in listening to your cat's

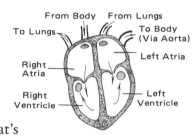

SCHEMATIC DRAWING OF HEART

From Body   From Lungs
To Lungs
To Body (Via Aorta)
Left Atria
Right Atria
Right Ventricle
Left Ventricle

STETHOSCOPE heart, but one is not necessary to deal with everyday health problems you may encounter. The normal heart beats about one hundred ten to one hundred thirty times per minute in the resting cat. You can feel the heart beat by placing your fingertips or the palm of your hand against your cat's chest just behind the point of the elbow. Placing your hand completely around the lower part of the chest with your fingers on one side and your thumb on the other is another simple and easy way to feel

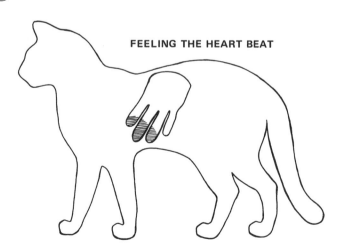

FEELING THE HEART BEAT

your cat's heart beat. If you cannot feel the heart beat, you can usually hear it by placing your ear (or a stethoscope) against the chest. Each heart beat consists of a strong, low-pitched thud followed by a less intense, higher pitched thud, followed by a pause—lub-dup. . .lub-dup. . .lub-dup.

To take your cat's pulse, place your fingers at the middle of the inside surface of the rear leg near the point where the leg meets the body. This is the area where the femoral artery passes near the skin allowing you to feel the pulse. The heart rate and pulse rate should, of course, be the same. It is easiest to count the heart rate or pulse for fifteen seconds then multiply by four to calculate the rate per minute.

FEELING THE PULSE

A measure of capillary circulation is *capillary filling time*. To measure this, press one finger firmly against your cat's gums. When you lift it away you will see a pale area which should refill with blood almost instantaneously. This measure of circulatory effectiveness can be helpful in evaluating possible shock (see page 169).

Blood is the fluid transported by the circulatory system. Blood consists of plasma, platelets, red blood cells and white blood cells. The composition of the liquid portion of the blood, *plasma*, is very complex. It carries nutrients throughout the body, removes wastes, including carbon dioxide, and provides a means of transport for the hormones produced by the endocrine glands, as well as transporting the particulate blood constituents. *Platelets* are produced primarily in the bone marrow of the adult cat.

37

These small bodies help prevent hemorrhage when a blood vessel is injured by aggregating together to form a physical barrier to blood flow and by stimulating clot formation. *Red blood cells* carry oxygen to the tissues and to a much lesser degree transport carbon dioxide away. They give blood its red color. There are several kinds of *white blood cells*, and each type has a particular function. As a group the white cells are most important in preventing and fighting infection. The red blood cells and white blood cells are often changed in numbers and types circulating when a cat becomes sick. The measurement of these cells by means of a *complete blood count* performed by your veterinarian is frequently necessary for correct diagnosis and treatment of cat health problems.

The *spleen* is an abdominal organ which, although not necessary for life, has many functions related to the blood. You may have felt this organ during your examination of the digestive system (see page 26). In the adult cat the spleen is a site for the production of some white cells and, in times of need, it can produce red cells as well. It is a blood reservoir which can supply large numbers of red cells rapidly when the body needs oxygen. The spleen also removes old and abnormal red blood cells from circulation and stores some red cell components, such as iron.

The *lymph nodes* are important structures which are responsible for the production of a special kind of white blood cell called the *lymphocyte* and which are important in protecting the blood from invasion by foreign agents such as bacteria traveling in the lymph paths. For more information about the lymph nodes and lymphocytes see pages 76 and 165.

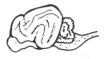 **Nervous and Endocrine Systems**

The integration of the functions of the various parts of the body is the main function of the nervous system and of the endocrine system. You cannot normally see or feel any of the components of these systems when you examine your cat. Nonetheless, if one system or the other is functioning abnormally it is usually not long before some striking change will occur in your animal. In general, the *nervous system* (brain, spinal chord and peripheral nerves) is responsible for rapid body adjustments to environmental and internal stimuli. The *endocrine system* for the most part is responsible for more gradual responses which are mediated by chemical substances secreted by endocrine glands into the blood stream *(hormones)*. Complete neurological and endocrine examinations are not a routine part of your or your veterinarian's physical exams. For your information a brief outline of the functions of the various endocrine glands is listed on the next page. Look at the drawings of the internal anatomy to see where these various glands are located. For very detailed information about these glands and other parts of your cat's anatomy and physiology, you may want to consult the following books:

Gilbert, Stephen G., *Pictorial Anatomy of the Cat*, University of Washington Press, Seattle, Washington.

Swenson, Melvin J., ed., *Dukes' Physiology of Domestic Animals*, Cornell University Press, Ithaca, New York.

Ganong, W.F., *Review of Medical Physiology*, Lange Medical Publications, Los Altos, California. (A human physiology text, but the information for the most part applies to cats.)

Don't be surprised if your first examination of your cat takes an hour or two. If you have a kitten or an adult cat that has not been handled frequently before, it may take a full day to complete the exam because you may have to divide it into several parts separated by rest periods to compensate for their reluctance to hold still for examination. Repeat your physical examination at least once a week while you are learning what is normal for your cat. By doing this you will train your cat to cooperate and you will soon find that you no longer need to refer to this book so often. The time it

Endocrine Gland	Function
Pituitary-Hypothalamus	Regulates the activity of ovaries, testes, thyroid and adrenal cortex. Secretes growth hormone which stimulates growth of body tissues. Controls milk secretion and milk let down. Affects body water balance.
Thyroid	Controls metabolic rate, affects calcium and phosphorus metabolism.
Parathyroids	Influence calcium and phosphorus metabolism.
Adrenals	Cortex: Influences carbohydrate, protein, electrolyte metabolism. Medulla: Secretes adrenalin, noradrenalin which help body prepare for emergencies.
Testes	Influence development of masculine characteristics, influence sex drive.
Ovaries	Influence development of feminine characteristics, influence sexual behavior, estrus, pregnancy.
Islet cells of pancreas	Secrete insulin, glucagon which affect blood sugar level.
Kidney	Renin: Affects blood pressure. Erythropoietin: Stimulates red cell production.
Cells of digestive tract	Secrete various hormones which regulate digestive tract motility and secretion of digestive enzymes. Some control over insulin secretion.
Pineal body	Exact function unknown; may affect sexual development and sexual cycles.

takes for you to perform the examination will shorten considerably as you practice. You should eventually be able to finish it in about fifteen minutes. Most veterinarians become so skilled at physical examination that, until you become aware of what they are doing, you may not even realize that a physical examination is being performed. Your veterinarian may easily perform a routine physical in five or ten minutes. Special examinations, of course, take much longer.

Once you are familiar with your cat's anatomy, how frequently you repeat certain parts of a physical examination varies. You can get a good idea of your cat's general health daily by just being aware of their appetite and activity. Be sure to examine the ears, eyes, teeth, and skin at least every two weeks. And examine the mammary glands of females, in particular, monthly. If your cat spends a considerable portion of their time outside, you will probably have to make more of a conscious effort to do the examinations. Be sure to set aside several times a week to study your cat's condition; most illnesses are best treated if discovered early.

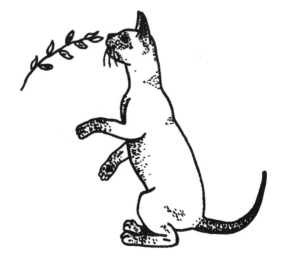

Preventive Medicine —
How to Care for a Healthy Cat

Training
Grooming
Nutrition
Traveling With or Shipping a Cat
Preventive Vaccination Procedures
Internal and External Parasites

Preventive Medicine Calendar

Daily: Feed a balanced diet. See page 58.

Groom cat as demanded by coat type and cat's habits. See page 50.

Observe cat's general external appearance, attitude, activity and appetite. Any change may indicate a need for complete physical examination.

Clean litter pan, observe cat's stool and, if possible, also observe the urine. (For outdoor cats, look for evidence of abnormal stool on coat.)

Weekly: Examine for external parasites and treat as necessary. See pages 95 through 103.

Examine ears. See page 53.

Clean teeth if your cat's teeth demand it. See page 56.

Administer hairball preventive. See page 150.

Every two weeks: Check claw length and appearance and trim, if necessary. See page 54.

Examine teeth if weekly cleaning is not necessary. See page 27.

Monthly: Examine mammary glands. See page 19.

Bathe, if necessary. See page 50.

Every six months: Perform a complete physical examination if one has not been indicated earlier.

Take a fecal sample to a veterinarian, particularly if there is an internal parasite problem in your area. See page 83.

Yearly: Take your cat to a veterinarian for a physical examination and booster vaccinations as necessary. See page 76.

Preventive Medicine

Preventive medicine is the best kind of medicine. Your veterinarian practices it when they vaccinate your cat for certain communicable diseases (see page 76). You can practice it by giving your cat good regular care at home, as discussed in this section. If you practice preventive medicine regularly, the occasions when your cat will need the care of a veterinarian can often be limited to yearly physical examinations and booster vaccinations. In the long run, preventive medicine is most economical, both financially and in terms of the stresses placed on your cat's body.

Indoor vs. Outdoor Cats

One of the best things you can do in terms of preventive medicine for your cat is to keep them inside. This applies particularly to city cats and to cats which live in neighborhoods heavily populated with other cats, dogs, and people. Strict enclosure is not necessary; a system whereby your cat spends most of their time indoors and is supervised outdoors is just about as satisfactory in health terms. However, do not allow your cat to roam without restriction, or purposely force your cat outdoors if you would like to avoid frequent trips to the veterinarian. Also be sure to provide your cat with a safe collar and an identification tag if they are to be allowed outdoors. Indoor cats and cats that stick close to home when outdoors miss out on nothing necessary for a happy, healthy life, and experience infectious disease, automobile accidents, poisoning, gun-shot wounds and cat fights much less frequently than their roaming peers.

45

Make the decision as to whether your cat is to have free access to the outdoors early in their life, then stick to it. Cats kept indoors when young usually show little desire to roam, even when allowed outside later in life.

Training

The training necessary to make a cat easy to live with is minimal when compared to what the average dog must be taught in order to make it a pleasant companion. Training for many cats includes only housebreaking and an incidental learning to respond to their name, but many other things can and, sometimes, must be taught. Some cats shake hands, retrieve balls, sit on command, and do other tricks that are amusing, but not necessary to being a good companion. Since only a small part of this book is devoted to understanding your cat's behavior and modifying it when necessary, you may find the following book interesting and useful:

Fox, M.W., *Understanding Your Cat*, Coward, McCann & Geoghegan, Inc., New York, 1974.

Teaching A Cat Their Name   Use your cat's name frequently during training. Be sure to use it at pleasurable times such as at feeding, play and while being petted, as well as to get your cat's attention before correction. If you are consistent in its use, your cat will learn their name quickly. And if you associate it with only "good" things, your cat will soon come running in response to their name with no special effort.

Punishment   Although many cats do not seem to respond to punishment as correction for misdeeds, many others do. Each time you get a cat you will have to determine what method is best for that individual. In general, try to avoid physical punishment, while getting your cat to respond to gentle words and petting. Use a sharp "No!" when you find your cat doing something undesirable and see if this is sufficient to stop the behavior and prevent its recurrence. If harsh words

46

and praise are not sufficient you may have resort to picking your cat up by the scruff and shaking them or to a spank on the rump. (One caution: never punish your cat after they come in response to their name. They may think you are punishing them for coming!) Cats are intelligent creatures, however, and this type of physical punishment sometimes results in a cat who will "behave" when you are around, but immediately do the undesirable when you leave the room or the house. A squirt from a water gun or spray bottle will often work better than more direct punishment. Keep a filled weapon at hand. When your cat chews on your plants, gets into the fireplace, climbs on the curtains or does something equally irritating in their explorations, squirt them. Their undesirable behavior will usually stop after a few corrections and the squirt gun method often produces long lasting results.

Toys

Be sure to provide your cat with sufficient diversions of their own. Continued correction will not result in a "perfectly behaved" cat if you fail to provide permissible amusements. Many commercial cat toys are good, but be sure to inspect them well before assuming they are safe. All cats' toys should be big enough to prevent swallowing them (even with difficulty) and should be sturdy enough to prevent them from being torn apart and eaten. Avoid string and thread and also balls of yarn if your cat unrolls them and chews on the yarn. Cats often swallow these materials, which can cause serious gastrointestinal problems. A patch of fresh catnip, catnip toys, paper bags, empty thread spools, stuffed socks and bones which can be chewed on but not swallowed are good inexpensive toys that many cats enjoy. A cloth-covered cat "tree" is more expensive, but is often immediately adopted as a favorite perch and scratching area instead of furniture. (For more information about scratching posts see page 54.)

Age to Get A Kitten

If you have a choice, probably the best time to bring home a new kitten is when they are between seven to ten weeks of age. Although a critical period for socialization has not been firmly established for the cat as it has for the dog, there is evidence that kittens which do not receive normal

47

contact with other cats when young (before six weeks of age) tend to develop abnormal behavioral patterns, such as extreme shyness or aggressiveness, and may never relate well to other cats. By waiting until your cat is seven to ten weeks of age to bring them home you allow time for proper social interaction with their littermates and mother, proper weaning, and, usually, training to a litter pan, while still acquiring a kitten young enough to be able to adapt well to you and to their new environment in your home.

Unless you want to share your bed with your cat, give your kitten a place of their own from the first night you have them home. Get a cat bed or use a cardboard box and line it with a clean, washable towel or blanket. Place this bed in your cat's special area. If your kitten does not yet know how to use a litter pan, it is probably best to choose an area which is large enough to contain your kitten's bed, their food and water dishes, and a litter pan and enclose the kitten in at night (and whenever you must leave the house) to avoid toilet accidents on the floor. If your kitten is already using a litter pan, a barricade is probably not necessary; just be sure the pan is within easy reach and the bed is in a warm and draft-free area. Be firm and be consistent with this arrangement if you plan not to share your bed with your cat. It's easy to take a charming, tiny kitten to bed for a few nights; it's just about impossible to keep an adult cat off a cozy bed once they have claimed it as their own.

Housebreaking   Because cats are instinctively fastidious about where they eliminate, housebreaking the average cat is usually very easy. Often a kitten will already be using a litter pan when you first bring them into your home. If not, you will probably be able to train your cat to use one very quickly.

Get a smooth-surfaced pan (plastic or enamel-surfaced ones are usually best) which can be easily cleaned and disinfected; or use disposable litter boxes. Newspapers, sawdust or wood shavings are sanitary materials to use for litter, but I think commercial clay litters are best. They are clean, absorbent, tend to reduce odors and most cats seem to like them. Line the pan with the litter material, then put it in a place easily accessible to your cat. If you have a kitten, be sure they don't have to go too far to find the litter pan at first and be sure the sides of the pan aren't too high to climb over easily or you may have trouble with housebreaking. If your cat uses the litter pan correctly from the start, great. If not, you can help them learn the proper behavior by placing them into the pan after eating, when they awaken and after play. Praise them when you see the desired results and correct them when they begin to eliminate in the wrong place by saying "No!" sharply and firmly and placing them in the litter pan to finish.

If you choose to allow your cat free access to the outdoors, you can use the litter pan to finish the housebreaking process. Once your cat has become accustomed to going in and out, move their litter pan gradually from its original site toward their usual exit. If at any time during this procedure your cat does not use the pan, move it back to the last place for a day or two before continuing on. In a few days your cat should be using their pan right next to the exit. Then move the pan to a place just outside the exit. After your cat has been using the pan outside for a few days, remove it entirely. Most cats will continue to choose to eliminate outside. However, cat feces in the garden can be a human health hazard (see page 83). If your cat uses your garden as their toilet, use gloves while gardening or at least wash your hands thoroughly afterwards. And don't allow children, whose habits tend to be less sanitary, to play in areas where your cat may bury their stools.

Remove stools from the litter pan daily. This is best accomplished with a spoon-like litter strainer which can be purchased at a pet store or supermarket. If you use disposable litter pan liners or completely disposable litter pans, discard them at least every fourth day. Otherwise wash the litter pan thoroughly every fourth day. (Do this outdoors or in a sink not used for washing dishes or bathing.) Use hot water, soap and chlorine bleach, then rinse the pan well and allow it to dry before replacing the litter. DO NOT use disinfectants containing phenol (carbolic acid), cresols, resorcinol or hexyresorcinol; they can be toxic to cats. If this cleaning schedule is not sufficient to keep odors at an

49

acceptable level, baking soda is a safe product you can try. Place a layer of it equal to about one third the weight of the litter in the bottom of the litter pan each time you change it.

Sometimes a litter pan acceptable to you won't be one acceptable to your cat. Most cats do not like wet or dirty litter pans and will begin to eliminate in abnormal places when dissatisfied with their normal toilet area. So be sure to remove litter from the pan and replace soiled with fresh material whenever it becomes wet, even if this occurs more frequently than your normal cleaning schedule. Elimination in abnormal places may also occur when the litter pan is clean and dry. Sometimes this is because you have changed litter materials after using one kind for a long period of time. Be sure to check the litter pan situation if you find stool or urine in abnormal places around the house once your cat has been housebroken. And for more information on elimination in undesirable places see pages 150, 156 and 161.

Grooming

Whether you will need to follow a particular grooming schedule with your cat will depend greatly upon the length and density of their coat, whether they spend the majority of their time indoors or outdoors, and whether they groom themselves well. In general, outdoor cats will need baths and brushing more frequently in order to make them pleasant companions than cats spending all their time indoors. Indoor cats may need their nails trimmed frequently. Read this section and decide for yourself which grooming schedule you need to apply to your cat.

Bathing
Although cats groom themselves, not all do it sufficiently often or sufficiently well to keep themselves clean enough to be pleasant companions and have a healthy and good-looking haircoat and skin. Tomcats who spend a great deal of time outside seem to be the worst offenders, but any cat may need a bath on occasions when they become

dirty, or for other health reasons. Accustom your cat to bathing early in life so it won't be difficult to do later when the necessity arises. I think it is best to give a young cat a bath about once a month starting around three months of age, just so they become adjusted to the bathing procedure. But you can bathe a kitten as young as seven or eight weeks if you do it quickly and prevent the possibility of their chilling. Bathing itself does not cause illness, but the stress of being chilled can predispose any cat, particularly a young one, to disease. Once your cat has become familiar with bathing and is cooperative, use their appearance, feel and odor as guides to bathing frequency. Once a month is usually sufficient for an average cat with healthy skin. *When To Start Baths*

How Often To Bathe

Unless your cat has a specific skin problem requiring medicated shampoos recommended by a veterinarian, use a good quality cat shampoo or a gentle human shampoo (e.g., baby shampoo) for bathing. Avoid bar soap and dishwashing detergents since they seem to be particularly drying and very irritating to some cats' skin and hair. A creme rinse (human or for pets) can be used following shampooing to make the comb-out of long-haired cats easier. *Shampoo To Use*

Before the bath it is a good idea, but not absolutely necessary, to protect your cat's ear canals and eyes from the soap and water. This can be done by placing large wads of cotton firmly inside the ears and by applying a gentle ophthalmic ointment, petrolatum, or a drop of mineral oil into each eye. Long-haired cats should be combed out before bathing to make grooming afterwards easier. *How To Bathe*

Place your cat in a sink or bathtub and use warm water. If your cat is an adult and a little uncooperative, gain control of them and avoid scratches to yourself by grasping them with one hand around the base of the head just behind the ears or by the scruff of the neck (see page 204). Then use your free hand for soaping and rinsing. If your cat is extremely insecure, a soft rope looped around their neck and tied to a fixture (never a hot water faucet) will keep them in the tub. But never leave a cat tied in this manner alone. Better than this though is a window screen placed in the tub. Most cats will cling to this with their claws, remaining in the

51

tub and leaving you both hands free for the job at hand. Praise your cat if they are cooperative, and try to correct them with a "No" if they are not. As a last resort, your veterinarian can provide tranquilizers to use when it is necessary to bathe an extremely unmanageable cat.

Start the bath by wetting your cat thoroughly, then apply the shampoo and suds it up. Two shampoo applications may be necessary if your cat is very dirty. Then follow the sudsing with a thorough rinsing, since any soap left on the skin can be irritating and any stunned parasites (see page 95) left on the skin may wake up later and continue their activities. Apply a creme rinse now, if you are using one, then rinse again thoroughly. Towel drying is usually sufficient, but, if you accustom your cat to the sound, you can use a drier for human hair to speed the drying process.

Grooming Between Baths

The kind of grooming your cat's coat needs between baths depends on its length and character. Short-haired cats usually need little grooming, but you may want to give them a bi-weekly brushing to distribute the oils and to remove loose hair, lessening the amount you find around the house and the amount they ingest while self-grooming. A grooming mitt works well for this. Long-haired cats usually need frequent (preferably daily) brushing to prevent matted coats and to lessen the

Hair Mats possibility of hairballs occurring (see page 150). Mats of hair often occur behind the ears and under the legs, so don't forget to brush or comb these areas well. When you find small mats, they can often be teased apart with a comb. If they become large, cut them away with scissors or clippers.

GROOMING MITT

Tar, Paint, Oil Tar, paint, and oil can be difficult substances to remove from the coat. DO NOT use gasoline, turpentine, kerosene, paint remover or other similar substances in an attempt to remove them. Cut out small accumulations of tar or paint. Large amounts of tar can be removed without cutting by soaking the affected hair in

52

vegetable or mineral oil for twenty-four hours (e.g., bandage tar covered feet soaked in oil), then washing with soap and water. Small patches of oil on the coat may be able to be removed by sprinkling them with constarch, allowing it to soak up the oil, then brushing it out. Large amounts can be treated with mineral oil as you would for tar. As a last resort (e.g., if your cat is covered with oil) use a detergent bath.

Skunk Odor

If your cat gets sprayed by a skunk, bathe them in soap and water, then follow with a tomato juice soak. Pour on the juice straight; let it sit for about ten minutes, then rinse it out.

Foxtails

In areas such as California where *foxtails* (wild barley) or other troublesome plant awns grow, longer-haired cats with access to the outdoors need to have their coats examined for them daily in the late spring, summer and fall. Although problems with plant awns are much less common in cats than dogs, because of cats' grooming habits, awns not discovered and removed, easily penetrate the skin causing irritation and infection.

Ears

Most cats who groom themselves well keep their ears extremely clean and need no help from you. Small accumulations of wax are normal. If your cat doesn't remove them you can do it easily following a bath by using a damp towel or soft cloth. Wrap the cloth over your index finger, then clean out the excess wax and dirt as far down the ear canal as your finger will reach. Any folds or crevices you cannot reach into with your finger can be cleaned using a cotton-tipped swab moistened with water or mineral oil. You cannot damage your cat's eardrums by cleaning in this manner unless you are extremely forceful, because the ear canals are very narrow and deep.

CLEANING EARS

A Cloth

A Cotton Swab

53

If your cat has an inflammation or infection of the ear *(otitis)* special ear cleaning may be necessary (see page 132).

Claws

As part of their inherited behavioral tendency to groom themselves cats condition their claws (toenails). This they do by scratching on objects which catch the outer, worn claw covering and remove it, exposing the sharp new claw beneath. Although this is a completely normal feline behavior, it can be a problem for owners with cats confined to the indoors, since if they are not provided with a scratching post or board, cats will use rugs, furniture and draperies for their scratching, damaging or ruining these furnishings completely. (Cats also remove their worn outer claw coverings with their teeth, but this is seen less frequently and doesn't cause problems for owners as does their scratching behavior.)

Provide your cat with a scratching post or board while they are very young in order to avoid problems later. You can use commercial scratching posts—horizontal or vertical posts usually covered with carpet—or you can make a scratching post yourself. A board about eight inches wide and a foot to a foot and one-half long, bare or fabric covered, can be attached to the wall. It should be at a height such that your cat can rest comfortably on their rear feet while scratching, so it may have to be moved as your cat grows. A good scratching post can be made of a bare or fabric-covered board built freestanding horizontally or vertically as well. Many cats seem to prefer a log with the bark still on it.

Place the scratching object near your cat's sleeping or resting area when first beginning their training, because they usually tend to stretch and scratch just after awakening. Then praise and pet them whenever they use it. Whenever your cat scratches at furniture or other undesirable objects, correct them and take them to their scratching post. With consistency and repetition your cat should soon be using their scratching post and leaving other objects alone.

If you have an adult cat that you have failed to

condition to a scratching post while young, your problem may be more difficult. The basic principles of correction and praise are the same, but it may take much longer for you to achieve the desired results. Try to provide a scratching post covered with a material at least as desirable as the things they have been scratching on before or you may not get far at all. At least one behaviorist feels that fabrics with longitudinally-oriented threads are preferred, but you may have to experiment a little before finding just the right one. During the training period you may have to trim your cat's nails in order to avoid furniture damage.

Trimmers for human nails are satisfactory for trimming cats' claws or you may use nail trimmers designed especially for pets, such as the White's type. To trim your cat's nails, extend the claw as described on page 14. If you do this in good light and your cat's nails are not darkly pigmented, you will be able to see the pink *dermis* (quick). Cut the nail just beyond the point where you see the dermis end. If you cut into the dermis, it is painful to the animal and some bleeding will usually occur. The bleeding stops, but the pain will make your cat reluctant to have a nail trim the next time. Pigmented nails are harder to trim although with good light you can often see the quick in these as well. If you can't see the dermis, the easiest rule to follow is to cut the nail just beyond the point where it starts to curve downward. If you accidentally trim the nail into the quick and the bleeding doesn't seem to be stopping, you can apply a styptic pencil, Monsel's solution (ferric subsulfate, available from pharmacists) or you can bandage the foot firmly for about an hour (see page 207).

If you have accustomed your cat to handling at a young

How To Trim Claws

"WHITE'S" NAIL TRIMMER

X-SECTION OF CLAW

Claw Ungual Process

Trim Here

3rd Phalanx

2nd Phalanx

Pad

55

age, nail trimming should be a one person job. If your cat seems particularly disagreeable, try to accustom them to the procedure gradually, trimming a few nails at a time and correcting them for bad behavior before resorting to a second person for aid.

Declawing
Declawing *(onchyectomy)* is a surgical procedure which can be resorted to when nail trimming and attempts to train a cat to use a scratching post have failed. It may also be necessary for cats which are not careful to keep their claws sheathed during play. It should not, however, become a routine procedure for pet cats. It is too painful a procedure to be performed unnecessarily and cats who have been declawed are at a disadvantage in some situations. They are unable to protect themselves well against dogs or other cats, and often cannot climb as well as normal cats to escape danger. Therefore, declawed cats should not be allowed outdoors unsupervised. When you and your veterinarian agree that declawing is necessary, the surgery is performed under general anesthesia in the veterinary hospital. The front claws are removed completely so regrowth is impossible and the feet are usually bandaged for forty-eight hours. The rear claws can be removed if desired, but this is unnecessary since they do not usually cause a problem in scratching behavior or accidental injury to the cat's owner during play and are necessary for a cat to scratch themselves. Once the bandages are removed, your cat will be able to return home and within two weeks should be free from pain.

Teeth

Almost all cats need special attention given to their teeth to preserve them and to minimize mouth odors. Most
Tartar

cats, like most people, develop deposits called dental *tartar* or *calculus* on their teeth. When present it is most obvious on the premolar and molar teeth as a hard yellow-brown or grayish-white deposit which cannot be removed by brushing or scraping with a fingernail. Its presence is not normal (see page 27). It can cause gum disease *(gingivitis, periodontitis)* which is accompanied by discomfort and can eventually lead to loss of teeth. Many cats develop mouth disease and lose teeth. Most do not develop cavities, but lose teeth because their owners miss the early stages of gum disease.

Once tartar is present it can only be removed properly Tartar with special instruments, either tartar scrapers or an Prevention ultra-sonic tooth cleaner. Tartar is best removed by a veterinarian, but if you would like to learn to do it at home, your veterinarian will probably be willing to show you how. Tartar originates from a soft white to yellow-colored substance on teeth called *materia alba* or plaque which is material left on the teeth after eating. You can remove this plaque and prevent tartar formation in the following ways:

1) Feed your cat a large proportion of their diet as dry cat food. Although feeding a hard food diet will not absolutely prevent tartar in all cats, because its formation is dependent on conditions in each cat's mouth, it has been shown experimentally that, in general, cats eating an all-dry food diet accumulate substantially less tartar and have much less plaque than cats eating solely a moist, soft food.

2) Encourage your cat to chew on (but not eat and swallow) large, hard bones. This will help remove plaque by abrasion. Although most cats will not chew on hard rubber toys or rawhide toys as dogs will, if you give them large hard bones with a little meat on them when they are young, cats will often develop the habit of bone chewing. Beef and lamb marrow bones are good. Avoid bones which splinter, such as pork chop and chicken bones.

3) Clean your cat's teeth yourself once or twice a week. You can use a toothbrush, but a gauze pad or rough cloth works as well. Moisten it with water, then scrub the teeth and gums vigorously. It's not necessary to do the inner tooth surfaces, because the motion of the tongue keeps the areas next to it relatively free from plaque.

CLEANING THE TEETH

If your cat's gums bleed even though they look healthy otherwise, it is not usually because you have scrubbed too hard, but because

57

they are in the early stages of disease. Good tooth care should cause an early problem to correct itself. If you see loose teeth, that the gums are red and pulling away from the teeth (receding), or if bleeding gums do not improve with good preventive care as suggested above, you probably will need the help of a veterinarian to clear up the condition. You can begin treatment at home with a daily gum massage. Use your finger, bare or wrapped in a cloth, or use a cotton-tipped swab. Make gentle circular motions while pressing firmly against the gums.

Nutrition

General Information About Feeding

Cats meet their nutritional requirements by ingesting proteins, fats, carbohydrates, vitamins and minerals just as people do. Unlike for people and dogs, however, minimum requirements for all the necessary food substances have not yet been well established for cats. So the task of providing a proper diet during growth, adulthood and old age, as well as at times of special nutritional needs, can be difficult. Always keep in mind that often it is only after months (or years) of nutritional deprivation that signs of disease may appear and that the effects of inadequate nutrition can usually never be reversed. To help you keep up with the latest developments in feline nutrition, the following publication (which is frequently revised) may be of use:

National Research Council, *Nutrient Requirements of Laboratory Animals*, National Academy of Sciences, Washington, D.C., 1972.

Proteins

Proteins are essential substances for growth and repair. They cannot be synthesized in the body from dietary constituents other than protein; therefore, they are extremely important to nutrition. Proteins are composed of amino acids and can vary widely according to the kinds of

58

amino acids present and their proportions. *Essential* amino acids cannot be synthesized in the cat's body and must be supplied by the diet in special proportions if they are to be used optimally. Proteins which supply the essential amino acids in near optimum quantities are given a high *biological value* because they can be used efficiently by the body. Proteins with a high biological value are the best ones to feed and the best upon which to base commercial diets since they are most economical in terms of body work and more economical on a pound for pound basis than proteins which cannot be used so completely when fed alone. Examples of proteins assigned a high biological value are eggs, milk, fish meal, muscle meat, soybeans and yeast.

Diets providing about thirty-four to forty percent protein on a dry weight basis from mixed sources have been found to be adequate to meet the protein requirements of growing kittens' while protein levels of twenty-five percent are generally sufficient for adult maintenance. These levels are necessary to meet a protein requirement for cats which has been estimated to be anywhere from two to four times that for dogs at equivalent growth stages. These high requirements for proteins make it obvious that for at least this one reason—protein content—rations designed for dogs are not adequate for cats.

Eggs are an excellent source of protein for use as a diet supplement. If you feed eggs frequently, however, they should be cooked. Egg white is not digested as well raw as when cooked, and raw egg white contains a substance called *avidin* which binds *biotin* (a B vitamin), interfering with its absorption from the gut. Although the biotin requirement for cats has not been established, I think the best policy to follow is one which safely insures the supply of the most vitamins possible. Raw egg yolks may be fed if separated from the whites.

Milk and milk products such as cottage cheese or yogurt are also good protein sources and good sources of calcium and phosphorus as well. Some cats, however, develop diarrhea when fed any milk products. Others may develop diarrhea only when fed large amounts of them. Diarrhea associated with the ingestion of milk products occurs when *lactose* (milk sugar) is not digested. Undigested lactose attracts water into the intestine causing diarrhea, so provide milk and milk products as supplements to your cat's diet with care. If loose stools develop when milk is fed, stop it immediately and wait for the stool to return to normal before trying new milk products. Cats which cannot drink milk without developing diarrhea can often eat yogurt, which has a much lower lactose content.

Fats   Fats provide the most concentrated source of energy (nine Calories per gram) of any of the necessary dietary components. They carry fat soluble vitamins (A, D, E, K) and supply fatty acids (e.g., linoleic, linolenic) which are probably as necessary in cats as they are in other animals for healthy skin and hair. The fat content of a diet adequate for cats needs to be much higher than one adequate for dogs. Not only does a high proportion of fat in the diet improve palatability, but kittens fed a high fat ration (with optimal protein provided) grow better than those provided with diets lower in fats. Diets containing twenty-five to thirty percent fat are recommended. Most commercial dry foods and semi-moist foods fail to provide fat in optimal quantities for cats and should be supplemented with bacon fat, butter or cooking oils as follows: add four and one-half tablespoonsful of oil per pound dry food. Add three and one-half tablespoons oil per pound semi-moist food.

Carbohydrates   Carbohydrates (sugars, starch, cellulose) are used by the cat as energy sources, and, under normal metabolic conditions to help maintain the blood glucose (sugar) level. Because carbohydrates are readily available as energy sources, they "spare" proteins allowing them to be used for more important structural jobs in the body instead. Cellulose, a carbohydrate which is not digested by cats, provides necessary bulk for proper intestinal function.

Although carbohydrates have not been demonstrated to be required in the diet, they can be utilized by cats as energy sources, particularly after being cooked (e.g., cereal grains, potatoes and certain other vegetables). If adequate levels of fat and protein are provided, carbohydrates may be present

60

up to thirty-three percent of the diet (or slightly more) and are used well.

Cats require about one ounce (thirty milliliters) of water per pound of body weight daily. They obtain this water in the food they eat and the liquids they drink. Water is also a by-product of metabolism; fat metabolism, in particular, is of great importance. The importance of foods in supplying the water requirements of cats is so great, in fact, that a cat on a moist food diet (which contains about 75% water) can easily be thought not to drink at all. Cats on other diets, however, do drink frequently and the actual amount of liquid a cat must drink daily is influenced by many factors in addition to diet, among them exercise, environmental temperature and the presence of fever, vomiting or diarrhea. So the best solution to the problem of water intake is to be sure that your cat has access to clean water at all times. (Milk may be provided as an additional water source if it does not cause diarrhea.) Do not give your cat water considered unfit for human consumption, and, if for some reason you are unable to give your cat free water access, be sure to offer water at least three times a day.

A cat can go without food for days and lose thirty to forty percent of their normal body weight without dying, but a water loss of ten to fifteen percent can be fatal. When cats stop eating (as they do frequently when sick) they must drink more water to make up for the decrease in intake in food and in the amount provided by metabolism and for possible increases in need. Turn to page 199 to find out about providing water for your cat during illness.

Although the required levels of all the essential vitamins which should be included in cats' diets have not been fully established, certain facts regarding the importance of various vitamins in the cat's diet have been established and should be heeded. The table on page 63 shows the currently recommended vitamin allowances. Special cases are discussed below.

Cats have a very high requirement for vitamin A in their diet as compared to dogs. Since they cannot convert *beta*-carotene (found in green vegetables) to vitamin A as do dogs, one must be sure that other sources of fully formed

61

vitamin A are provided in the diet to prevent a deficiency which can result in skin, eye, and reproductive changes. On the other hand, too much vitamin A in the diet can result in skeletal deformities and crippling.

In order to prevent vitamin A deficiency or excess, use a complete commercial cat diet with vitamin A added as a basis for feeding (see page 65) and use liver (high in vitamin A) only as a supplement for your cat's diet, not as a major part of it. Feed an adult cat no more than one ounce of beef liver twice weekly. If necessary, balanced vitamin-mineral preparations may also be used as dietary supplements to supply vitamin A. Use only ones recommended by your veterinarian and follow directions for use carefully.

Vitamin E   It is doubtful whether *under normal feeding conditions* vitamin E deficiency or excess will occur. There have been, however, many cases of vitamin E deficiency in cats. These have resulted from an abnormal feeding practice considered normal by poorly informed owners, usually the feeding of excessive quantities of red meat tuna. It has also occasionally followed the feeding of other fish diets, fish oils (e.g., cod liver oil) or large quantities of liver.

Pansteatitis   Vitamin E deficiency results in oxidation of body fat and its generalized inflammation called *pansteatitis* (steatitis). Its signs include lack of appetite, fever, and pain accompanied by reluctance to move. It can eventually end in death. Vitamin E deficiency should be diagnosed and treated by a veterinarian, but, more importantly, you can prevent its occurrence. Use a complete commercial cat food as your cat's basic diet and avoid frequent feeding of red meat tuna. Any tuna fed should be clearly marked—supplemented with vitamin E. Do not use fish oils (e.g., cod liver oil) as dietary supplements and feed liver only as previously recommended.

B Vitamins (Thiamine, Riboflavin, Pyridoxine, Pantothenic acid, Niacin, B_{12})   Cats have a very high requirement for the B vitamins. In most cases where requirements have been established, cats need (on a per kilogram basis) about twice the amount needed to keep a dog healthy. Since several B vitamins are destroyed by heating, such as that used during the processing of commercial cat foods, be sure complete diets you purchase are supplemented with B vitamins. Liver is high in B vitamins

62

(as well as vitamin A) so use it as recommended to help fulfill your cat's needs. Several B vitamins are synthesized by bacteria in a cat's intestines. This helps reduce the amount that must be obtained from outside sources. Intestinal conditions (e.g., diarrhea) can eliminate this internal source of B vitamins; therefore, during prolonged illnesses involving intestinal upset be sure to supplement the food.

Vitamin Requirements of the Growing Cat

Vitamin		Amt. Req. in Diet		Allowance Per Day Per Cat
		Dry (kg)	90% Dry	
A	IU/kg	27,777	25,000	1000-2000 IU
D	IU/kg	1,111	1,000	50-100 IU
E	IU/kg	151	136	0.4-4.0 mg
K	Requirements are very low. Probably synthesized in sufficient amounts by gut flora.			
B Vitamins				
Thiamine	mg/kg	4.4	4	0.2-1.0 mg
Riboflavin	mg/kg	4.4	4	0.15-0.2 mg
Pyridoxine (B6)	mg/kg	2.2	2	0.2-0.3 mg
Niacin	mg/kg	44	40	2.6-4.0 mg
Pantothenic acid	mg/kg	5.5	5	0.25-1.0 mg
Biotin	Requirements are very low. Probably synthesized in sufficient amounts by gut flora.			0.1 mg
Folic acid	Requirements are very low. Probably synthesized in sufficient amounts by gut flora.			
B12	Requirements not established.			
Choline	mg/kg	3,333	3,000	100 mg
Inositol	mg/kg	222	200	10 mg
C (Ascorbic acid)	Synthesized by the cat			

g =	gram, approximately 1/30 ounce
kg =	kilogram, one thousand grams, approximately 2.2. pounds
mg =	milligram, 1/1000 gram
IU =	international unit, a measure of vitamin activity. The amount in milligrams varies depending on the vitamin under consideration.

Minerals   Although the vitamin requirements of cats seem to be much higher than those for dogs, mineral requirements seem to be much lower (another reason to avoid feeding cats dog foods). Although few studies have been done that establish the mineral requirements of cats, it seems unlikely that a cat which eats a diet well-balanced in other respects would become deficient in minerals. Unsuspecting cat owners can more easily provide improper rather than inadequate mineral supplies for their pets. A good example of this problem is provided by the interrelationship among the minerals calcium and phosphorus and the vitamin D. These relationships are often upset by oversupplementation and/or by catering to a cat's food preferences instead of their needs.

Calcium,   Calcium and phosphorus should be present in the diet of *Phosphorus,* cats as ratio of about 1 to 1. If an adequate amount of each *Vitamin D* of these minerals is present, but the ratio is incorrect, abnormal mineralization of bone occurs in the growing kitten and in the adult cat as well. If adequate amounts of calcium and phosphorus in the proper ratio are provided, but without sufficient vitamin D, abnormalities of bone result again. Insufficient levels of vitamin D interfere with calcium absorption from the gut. Excessive amounts of vitamin D in the presence of adequate levels of calcium and phosphorus may result in excessive mineralization of bone, abnormal teeth and calcification of the soft tissues of the body. The delicacy of these relationships is apparent.

Unthinking or uninformed owners most often distort the calcium: phosphorus balance of their cat's diet by feeding an almost exclusively meat diet consisting of muscle meat, or organ meats such as liver, heart or kidney. All of these meats are almost devoid of calcium. So the calcium:phosphorus ratio being 1:15 or greater, prolonged feeding results in severe demineralization of bones, pain, and sometimes fractures or paralysis. An adult cat may exist on such a diet for years without showing signs of disease, but the bony changes are occurring nevertheless. A cat's requirements for vitamin D are low so that health problems relating to this nutrient are best avoided by preventing oversupplementation (see page 69). Remember that the wild ancestors and living relatives of the domestic cat rely on a wide variety of foods, including vegetable materials, to meet their nutrient requirements and feed your cat accordingly. Follow the dietary recommendations set out previously and on the following pages or follow the advice of a knowledgeable veterinarian to prevent nutrition-induced disease in your cat.

Choosing a Cat Food

Federal law requires that all cat foods carry a listing of their ingredients in decreasing order of their predominance in the ration. Other regulations require a guaranteed analysis listing minimum or maximum levels of certain food substances present (protein, fat, ash, water, carbohydrate). Unfortunately the required labels do not contain enough information to enable you to compare cat foods adequately with one another or to evaluate their nutritional quality. The guaranteed analysis gives no indication of the *quality* (digestibility or usefulness) of nutrients present nor does it give the exact quantities present. So you must rely on the companies themselves to produce a nutritious product for your cat. Companies are restricted from misrepresenting their products, however, and certain manufacturers have conducted research and feeding trials of their own in order to produce nutritious diets that need minimal supplementation. The following information will help you choose among commercial cat foods to find products to serve as a basic diet for your cat.

1) Diets for cats come in three forms: dry (about ninety percent dry matter), soft-moist (about sixty-five percent dry matter) and canned (about twenty-two to twenty-eight percent dry matter). In general, dry foods are the least expensive and the most well-balanced products to choose as bases for your cat's diet. Most cats eat these products well, particularly if they have been fed them since an early age. And, except for prescription cat foods available only through veterinarians, I think they are the best basic foods you can choose in terms of cost for quality. Their primary short-coming is in the fat content, which is usually

65

too low to meet the nutritional requirements of cats; so when they are fed fat should be added (see page 60).

Soft-moist foods are also in general basically sound diets in terms of their nutritional completeness. They tend to be expensive in comparison to dry foods and, along with dry foods, are generally deficient in fat. Humectants (moisture retainers) and preservatives, as well as high levels of sucrose make these products unsuitable for some cats who may develop digestive disturbances when fed them. Therefore, I think they are best used as a dietary supplement rather than as the primary part of a cat's diet.

Canned foods are generally the most expensive to feed. Complete canned foods can be excellent diets for cats, but if you choose such foods as your cat's basic diet, you must be very careful when reading package labels to be sure your cat is getting products intended to be complete diets and not dietary supplements. Canned products may consist of meat and meat by-products alone (unbalanced) or have cereal and/or vitamins and minerals added to make them balanced or complete rations for cats. If the label does not make it clear that the food is intended as a complete diet in itself, use the food only in addition to a wide variety of other foods and complete rations. Avoid canned foods in which large pieces or large proportions of bones, blood vessels or other undigestible material are present. In general, these are poor quality foods which are poorly utilized by your cat's digestive system.

When making a choice of cat foods among the three types available, be sure to compare them on a *dry weight basis.* Good quality products will generally have guaranteed analyses similar to those below.

Nutrient	Dry Food		Soft-moist		Canned meat type*		Canned Complete Ration Type	
	As Fed	Dry Basis	As Fed	Dry Basis	As Fed	Dry Basis	As Fed	Dry Basis
Protein	30%	34%	27%	40.9%	12%	54.5%	12%	42.8%
Fat	8%	9.1%	8.5%	12.9%	6%	27.2%	7%	25%
Carbohydrate	43%	48.8%	23.7%	35.9%	0.25%	1.1%	7%	25%
Ash	3.3%	3.8%	3.3%	5.0%	2.25%	10.2%	1.5%	5.4%
Fiber	4.0%	4.4%	3.5%	5.3%	1.5%	6.8%	0.5%	1.8%
Water	12%		34%		78%		72%	

*Canned meat type diets vary greatly in the quantities and quality of nutrients present. Water is the most constant element present.

2) Learn to distinguish complete from balanced rations. *Complete* rations have been tested by feeding trials and shown to be adequate to support life and promote reproduction when fed alone. *Balanced* rations, on the other hand, have not been subjected to the rigors of a feeding trial. They contain ingredients in quantities sufficient to meet the nutritional requirements of cats as recognized by the National Academy of Sciences. Unfortunately the nutrient requirements of cats have not yet been fully established; therefore, a balanced ration may not in itself be a sufficient diet for a cat. Be sure to read the labels thoroughly and choose a *complete* ration as a basic diet for your cat whenever possible. Balanced rations are probably acceptable if used in a varied feeding program (see page 68).

3) Look for a calcium:phosphorus ratio of approximately 1 to 1. Many cat foods contain enough information on their labels to enable you to determine the proportions of calcium and phosphorus present. To prevent calcium deficiency, avoid canned meat type products, in particular, if you cannot determine their calcium:phosphorus ratio.

4) Look for commercial cat foods which are supplemented with vitamins in their preparation. Important vitamins can be easily destroyed during processing and certain foods (e.g., meats) used in the preparation of cat rations are deficient in some vitamins to begin with. The best foods give you enough information on the package label to determine whether the product at least meets the known requirements. If such information is not listed look for vitamin A, E and B supplementation.

5) Consider the price. This particularly applies to canned foods. Cheap cat foods often contain cheap ingredients—poor quality protein and poorly digestible nutrients which pass through your cat unused. "Gourmet" type cat foods, on the other hand, may contain high quality ingredients but are often overpriced.

6) See what kind of effect the food has when eaten. If your cat gets diarrhea or becomes flatulent from a product, it probably should not remain part of their diet. Voluminous stools following the feeding of certain commercial foods

often indicate excessive amounts of fiber or other undigestible substances.

Feed A Varied Diet Once you have evaluated the commercial foods available as to their suitability as basic parts of your cat's diet, the next step is to actually formulate a diet for your cat. Complete foods which have undergone feeding trials should be adequate alone, but because expert nutritionists have not fully established the nutritional requirements of cats, it is probably best not to assume that any single commercial product will be adequate to fulfill all your cat's needs and best not to rely solely on cat food companies' honesty and expertise in evaluating feeding trials. Another reason not to use a single commercial food as the only means of feeding your cat is that cats develop narrow food preferences easily. Cats Are Not Finicky Eaters If you provide only one or a few kinds of food, or always indulge your cat in their favorite foods, they will often refuse to consume other nutritious foods and will tend to be reluctant to try new foods. This can easily lead to nutritional disease since it has been scientifically proven that cats given free choice of foods will not always select a diet that fulfills their nutritional requirements. Contrary to what advertisements would lead us to believe, *cats are not naturally finicky eaters and palatability is not an indication of the nutritional adequacy of a food.* Avoid producing nutritional inadequacies, imbalances and "picky eaters" by feeding a varied diet from the time your cat is very young. A nutritionally complete and adequately varied diet should resemble the following:

Feed Daily	Complete or balanced commercial dry cat food – add cooking oil (e.g., corn oil), butter or margarine at the rate of four and one-half tablespoonsful per pound fed. Feed once daily or allow free access.
	Complete or balanced canned foods – offer about one can per five pounds body weight. Canned foods containing less than five percent fat need fat added. Vary flavors frequently to avoid the development of food preferences and possible accompanying deficiencies.

68

Feed Twice A Week	Beef liver — one ounce per adult cat. Excessive liver feeding can produce vitamin A excess, diarrhea and dark-colored stools. Organ meats (spleen, heart, kidney) can be substituted for liver but fail to provide the high level of vitamins and minerals that liver does. Lightly cooking meat products helps prevent parasite transmission (see page 84, 86, 94) without destroying important vitamins.
Feed Occasionally	Cheese, yogurt, sour cream, milk, cooked vegetables, soups, cooked cereals, baby foods, brewers yeast, cooked clams or fish. (Some raw fish contains thiaminase, an enzyme which destroys thiamine and if fed to comprise more than ten percent of the diet may cause thiamine deficiency.) Cats may also have other "people foods" such as fruits, uncooked vegetables, sweets and condiments as treats if they do not cause digestive upsets; just remember that such foods do not contribute significantly to a cat's nutrition.

If you feed your cat a varied diet with good quality complete rations at its base, vitamin-mineral supplements are probably not necessary on a daily basis. In fact, over-supplementation can lead to nutritional diseases every bit as serious as those resulting from nutritional deficiencies. There are, however, times when balanced vitamin-mineral supplements which provide vitamins and minerals in proper amounts and proportions to meet known or estimated daily requirements can be beneficial to a cat's diet. Just remember to rely on balanced supplements available through your veterinarian or pet stores and to follow your veterinarian's or the package's instructions carefully. Avoid routine use of unbalanced dietary supplements such as bone meal, wheat germ or cod liver oil. Not only can such products be expensive, on a cost per unit nutrient basis, but unbalanced products may easily result in over-supplementation. Cod liver oil, for example, is a substance which is frequently misused as a dietary supplement for cats.

Vitamin-Mineral Supplements

One-half teaspoonful of N.F. cod liver oil contains about one hundred fifty-six I.U. of vitamin D. A mere teaspoonful of cod liver oil daily could result in vitamin D excess for a cat, accompanied by bone and soft tissue abnormalities, since the cat's requirement for this vitamin is low—no more than fifty to one hundred international units are recommended as a daily allowance.

Balanced vitamin-mineral preparations are probably best used to supplement the diet of sick (see page 199), pregnant or lactating (see page 240), or older cats (see page 184). I would also recommend them for any cat (growing or adult) which is not fed a varied diet similar to the sample one provided here.

Feeding a Kitten

In order to meet a kitten's nutritional requirements for proper growth and development you not only have to provide a diet that would be adequate to maintain an adult cat, but also provide about twice as many calories on a per pound body weight basis as for adults and thirty-six to sixty percent more protein as well. Frequent feedings will allow a kitten to meet the caloric requirement if the diet provided is well-balanced. Protein requirements are most easily filled by selecting complete commercial rations containing thirty-four percent or more protein on a dry weight basis and by using high quality protein foods to supplement the basic diet. Eggs, milk and milk products such as cottage cheese, sour cream and yogurt are high quality proteins which are valuable as dietary supplements for kittens. Be sure, however, to avoid any milk product which causes diarrhea when fed. Small amounts of cooked fish, muscle meat and beef liver (about one teaspoonful, 0.2 oz., per pound body weight per week) are also very good protein supplements which should be introduced at a young age along with other food permitted for adults (see page 68) to avoid the development of dietary preferences.

Changing A Kitten's Diet Be sure to find out what your kitten has been eating before you bring them home. If your kitten has not already been started on a well-balanced diet with quality complete foods as a basis, continue on their original diet for a day or two then gradually introduce the new foods that are to comprise the diet. Start with a single complete commercial cat food and add it to the original diet increasing the quantities of the new food gradually and decreasing the original until the kitten is consuming the new diet well. Then introduce other new foods in small portions at one time to avoid digestive upsets.

Kitten milk replacers, such a KMR®, can be very helpful during the early stages of feeding a kitten. Mixed with commercial foods, they make them easier to chew. They mimic queen's (mother's) milk and are therefore usually readily accepted; they do not have the tendency to produce diarrhea as does cow's milk, and they provide well-balanced sources of nutrients for a growing kitten. Be sure, however, to provide your kitten with fresh water at all times whether or not liquids such as milk replacers or cow's milk are provided.

It is physically impossible for a small kitten to consume enough food at one sitting (even of the highest quality) to meet their daily caloric requirement. The most convenient method to assure yourself that your kitten is consuming enough to meet their caloric needs if a complete diet is provided is to allow self-feeding. In this method food is left out where the kitten has free access to it and is changed as necessary to keep it fresh. Most kittens do not overeat with this system and it may help prevent boredom. Self-feeding must be abandoned or the portions left out reduced if the cat tends to become too fat.

How Often To Feed

Scheduled feeding is the system whereby you provide your kitten with several meals daily. It usually results in a cat that is anxious and ready to eat at mealtimes making it easy for you to determine when their appetite is not normal. It can, however, result in a cat that is "too attuned" to food with a tendency to gorge at mealtime and a tendency to fatness. If you choose the scheduled feeding method, provide your kitten with four to five meals a day until twelve weeks of age, three meals a day until six months of age, then feed them twice daily.

A combination of self and scheduled feeding may be used as well as relying totally on one system or the other. Many people successfully leave out a variety of commercial

71

complete foods for their cat's free choice feeding and use supplementary foods as "treats" or scheduled meals.

You can use the caloric table as a rough guide to estimating your kitten's daily needs. Information on cat food packages can also be used as feeding guides. But remember, each cat is an individual and as such has individualized caloric requirements. Your kitten's (or adult cat's) appearance can be used as a gauge of the adequacy of the diet fed. Look at and feel your kitten. A glossy coat, free of dandruff, a steady weight gain, good health and activity are all signs that tend to indicate that an adequate diet is being fed. Poor growth, a poor coat or frequent illness *could* mean that your kitten's diet is inadequate.

If you are using scheduled feeding, each meal should comfortably fill the kitten. If their stomach is distended and taut following a meal, or if they vomit shortly after eating, they may be eating too much at one time. More frequent, smaller meals may be necessary.

Any dietary problems with kittens not quickly resolved at home (within twenty-four to thirty-six hours) should be discussed with a veterinarian. Because of their rapid growth, small size and relatively high metabolic rate, what sometimes appear to be minor dietary problems can cause kittens to develop severe illnesses quickly.

Age In Weeks	Daily Calorie Requirement Per Pound Body Weight
0-1	190
1-5	125
5-10	100
10-25	65
25-30	50
Adult (female or neutered male)	about 40 or less
Adult tomcat	50
Adult pregnant	50
Adult lactating	125

For calorie content of various types of foods see page 155 and 200.

Feeding An Adult Cat

Although most adult cats require around fifty Calories per pound body weight per day, each cat has their own individual requirements and package information can only be used as a guide to feeding. Active cats require more calories than sedentary ones; uncastrated males, in particular, require more calories than neutered ones. Obesity in most cats, as in most people, usually indicates that you are feeding too much. Use whatever feeding method seems most convenient for you and your cat as long as you provide all the nutrients your cat needs. Most cats seem happiest if provided with at least two scheduled meals daily, free access to food or a combination of free access and supplemental meals. Of course, free access to food will have to be limited if you notice your cat becoming overweight.

Feeding An Older Cat

Cats undergo aging changes as do humans and may require special diets for maximum health and activity in old age. In general, older animals require fewer calories per pound body weight than when they were young; the amount of food given must usually be decreased to avoid obesity as a cat ages. Body changes can result in decreased utilization of nutrients, and, additionally, intestinal absorption of nutrients may be impaired. There is then a rationale for using balanced vitamin-mineral preparations to supplement the older cat's diet. Certain conditions such as recurrent constipation (see page 151), heart or kidney failure which tend to occur more often in older animals require special diets. The presence of such conditions should be determined by a veterinarian, however, before any special diet is used.

For information on feeding during pregnancy and lactation see page 232 and page 239.

For information on feeding orphan kittens see page 243.

For information on feeding sick animals see page 198.

Traveling With or Shipping a Cat

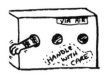

Accustom Your Cat To Travel Early

Although cats do not travel in automobiles with their owners as frequently as dogs do, trips to the veterinarian, to vacation spots or to new residences are frequent enough that real benefits are gained by accustoming your cat to travel when young. Not only are cats which become accustomed to riding and to confinement when young more relaxed with traveling, but they often come to enjoy it. Several cats I know have become seasoned travelers and companions which could be relied upon not to wander away from camp, because of their early training.

Take your cat on frequent short rides at first, then gradually lengthen them. Confine your cat to a carrier (particularly at first) while riding. This gives them a secure place of their own in which to ride and a portable refuge in strange places (e.g., hotel rooms, veterinarians' offices). It also prevents the annoying and sometime dangerous movements of a cat who is uneasy about traveling. Although you may eventually become confident that your cat will cause no problems when traveling, I think it is best to continue to confine your cat to a carrier while riding to avoid problems which might arise unpredictably.

Shipping On Commercial Carriers

The following items may help you when traveling with or shipping your cat on commercial carriers:

1) Airlines require a health certificate signed by an accredited veterinarian for shipping and other commercial carriers may also require one. Be sure to check with the shipper well before the departure date so you have time to obtain the necessary documents. Each state and foreign country has its own entry requirements for cats. Most states have no special requirements, but check with your veterinarian before traveling to be sure. Individual consulates are the best sources of current information for each foreign country.

2) Your veterinarian can prescribe safe tranquilizers for your cat if they seem particularly apprehensive about strange people and sounds. Some cats react unpredictably to tranquilizers, however, and become extremely wild and excitable. Cats accustomed to a carrier or traveling cage at

74

home before the trip (preferably while young) usually travel well without tranquilization, and I think this is most desirable. Special arrangements may often be made for a cat to travel with you in the passenger area, so investigate this possibility if you think your cat will travel poorly in baggage.

3) A traveling crate should be strong and have enough room to enable your cat to stand up, turn around, and lie down comfortably. A towel or other soft and familiar bedding can be placed inside as well as a small box containing litter, but these items are not absolutely necessary and on short trips often result in more mess than they're worth.

4) Attach an identification tag to *both* the crate and the cat stating the owner's name, the cat's name, the home address and the destination.

5) Do not feed the animal within eight hours prior to shipping.

6) Avoid giving water within about two hours of shipping time unless absolutely necessary (e.g., for health reasons, or high environmental temperature).

7) Do not place food or water in the crate. A *healthy* cat can go twenty-four hours without water, unless the environmental temperature is high, and much longer without food. If the trip is going to take longer than twenty-four hours (or if environmental temperature warrants it), be *sure* special arrangements are made for feeding, watering and exercise.

Preventive Vaccination Procedures

There are two major infectious feline diseases for which safe and effective vaccines are available — rabies and feline panleukopenia (feline enteritis, feline distemper). Each of these diseases can easily cause death in an unprotected cat. We are very fortunate to be able to prevent such serious illnesses with a procedure as technically simple as vaccination. (For more information on vaccines available for cats see page 139.)

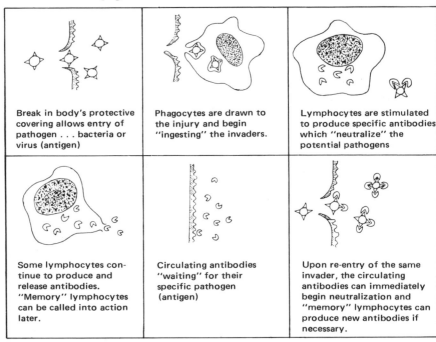

Break in body's protective covering allows entry of pathogen . . . bacteria or virus (antigen)	Phagocytes are drawn to the injury and begin "ingesting" the invaders.	Lymphocytes are stimulated to produce specific antibodies which "neutralize" the potential pathogens
Some lymphocytes continue to produce and release antibodies. "Memory" lymphocytes can be called into action later.	Circulating antibodies "waiting" for their specific pathogen (antigen)	Upon re-entry of the same invader, the circulating antibodies can immediately begin neutralization and "memory" lymphocytes can produce new antibodies if necessary.

How Vaccines Work

How Vaccines Work

Antigens are molecules that have particular areas on their surfaces which the body can recognize as "foreign." *Antibodies* are protein substances produced in the body which are responsible for recognizing these antigens. Antibodies are produced by cells called *lymphocytes* which originate in the bone marrow and multiply in the thymus, spleen and lymph nodes. When lymphocytes recognize that a foreign substance such as a virus or bacterium has entered the

76

body, they begin copious production of antibodies specific for the invader. Lymphocytes capable of antibody production against the invader multiply to produce progeny cells capable of producing more of the same antibodies. Some of these progeny cells go immediately into production of antibodies, others become resting cells which serve as the body's "memory" defense against a similar future invader. If the same (or a very similar) invader makes its appearance again at a later time, these cells are able to respond quickly to its presence.

Vaccination introduces a modified disease agent (antigen) into the body. Common methods of altering an organism's ability to produce disease are by killing it, and by "breeding" to an innocuous state. Modified viruses or bacteria are able to induce lymphocytes to produce antibodies capable of protecting the body against disease without actually producing the illness. Usually the body produces a higher (usually more protective) level of antibodies and antibodies most specific to a disease agent on the second exposure to a vaccine, but different vaccines vary in their ability to produce a protective antibody level on first exposure. The duration of the body's immunological memory for different viruses and bacteria also varies. These are two reasons why the number of original vaccinations necessary for protection and the frequency of booster vaccination vary with each disease.

Additional factors influence the vaccination of a young animal. Cats and dogs receive a small amount of antibody across the *placenta* (organ which communicates between mother and fetus before birth). They receive a much greater amount in the colostrum (first milk) and milk when they are nursing. It serves primarily to protect the kitten against disease for the first few weeks of life. Although kittens are capable of absorbing some antibodies through their gut for several days following birth, the first twenty-four hours are most important. Even if the kitten nurses adequately, however, whether or not they receive a protective level of antibody depends on how recently the mother was exposed to the disease in question or on how recently she was

Young Animals Are Special Cases

77

vaccinated, since the amount of antibody received against each particular disease is dependent on the level of circulating antibody in the mother. The antibody a kitten receives can be a disadvantage as well as being useful since it can cause interference with vaccination by tying up the vaccination-introduced antigen before it can stimulate the kitten's immune system. The protection kittens receive early in life against feline panleukopenia is an example.

Some kittens lose their protective immunity against panleukopenia acquired in nursing as early as six weeks of age, others as late as four months after birth. Therefore, the ideal vaccination schedule is individualized for each kitten if they are to be properly immunized. There are tests for determining the level of antibody against panleukopenia present in each kitten, but in general, they are too expensive and time consuming for routine use.

The techniques of vaccination are relatively simple. The knowledge of the proper handling of vaccines and of the physiology of the immune response is what makes it important to have a veterinarian interested in each animal as an individual vaccinate your cat. Vaccination by a good veterinarian also assures that your cat gets a physical examination when they are young, and then later as well to detect important changes that you may have missed. If a veterinarian vaccinates your cat without performing a thorough physical examination, something is wrong.

Feline Panleukopenia

Feline panleukopenia is an extremely common, very contagious, and often fatal viral disease which occurs in cats (both domestic and wild) and raccoons and other members of the raccoon family. Although this disease is commonly called *distemper,* it is *not* at all related to *canine distemper* which often occurs in young dogs. Other common names for panleukopenia are feline infectious enteritis, cat or show fever, and cat plague.

The incubation period (time from exposure to first signs of disease) for panleukopenia is usually about seven days, although it may vary from two to ten days. In young cats

78

(under six months) in particular, the disease can be so severe and of such rapid onset that death occurs before an owner is truly aware that signs of illness are present. More often the first signs are fever (frequently 104-105° F), listlessness, lack of appetite and vomiting usually accompanied by extreme dehydration. A cat may seem interested in drinking (some sit with their heads over or near their water bowls) but often will not drink or vomits soon after doing so. Diarrhea may accompany the first signs, but often seems to develop later. The stool is usually very watery and may contain pieces of intestinal lining and sometimes blood.

The procedure for initial immunization against pan- leukopenia varies depending, among other things, on the immune status of your kitten and on your ability to isolate your cat from exposure to the virus before vaccination is complete. Every effort should be made to keep your kitten away from cats which might be shedding the virus and away from panleukopenia-contaminated environments until vaccination is complete. The "panleuk" virus is shed in all bodily secretions and excretions and can be transmitted from cat to cat easily without bodily contact with the infected "carrier" cat. It is one of the most resistant viruses and can remain alive and a source of infection for susceptible cats for several months even after premises have been cleaned thoroughly. The best policy to follow is not to introduce a susceptible cat onto premises where a cat has had panleukopenia for three to four months following the episode. DO NOT allow an unvaccinated cat to associate with strange cats. Keep them indoors if necessary until vaccination is complete. Keep your kitten in your lap or in a carrier and out of contact with possibly sick cats while at your veterinarian's office.

Take your kitten to a veterinarian for their first vaccination at eight to ten weeks of age. A good veterinarian will perform a complete physical examination before administering the vaccine. At this time they will also be able to answer any questions you may have about the care of your cat. Don't be afraid to ask questions; no question is "dumb" and you may learn something very important by asking. The injection is usually given under the skin *(subcutaneously)* in

79

the back area between the shoulder blades and as with most vaccines, seems pretty painless; many kittens act as if they never realize they were vaccinated. Your veterinarian will ask you to bring your kitten back for a second vaccine in two weeks or more. In the meantime be sure to keep your kitten well isolated from exposure to disease. In general, two or three vaccinations are given before immunity is complete. Because there are various kinds of vaccines and variations in cats' ages at the time of first vaccination, fewer or more vaccinations may be necessary. The important thing to remember is that no matter how young when vaccination is begun a kitten should finish their vaccines *after* twelve to sixteen weeks of age. If you think the series is finished or have been told that the series is finished before your kitten is this age, bring them back to the veterinarian for another shot.

Treatment For Panleukopenia

If your cat contracts panleukopenia, it is important to have them examined by a veterinarian and to get intensive treatment started early. A complete blood count is necessary to help confirm the disease (the virus causes a marked decrease in the number of white blood cells present), and hospitalization is often necessary for its successful treatment. You may, however, be able to work with your veterinarian on treatment at home. Treatment consists of appropriate antibiotics, vitamins and supportive care including fluids, hand feeding, and antidiarrheal medication. Heroic measures such as blood transfusions have been necessary in some cases.

Although panleukopenia is often fatal, there is no reason to give up at the first sign of disease. Many cats have survived severe cases to live out normal, healthy lives.

Rabies

Rabies Affects The Nervous System

The rabies virus can infect any warm-blooded animal, including humans. It causes a disease of the nervous system manifested by changes in behavior preceding paralysis and death. The principal reservoirs of rabies in the United States are skunks, raccoons, bats and foxes. Bats and skunks may shed rabies virus in their saliva without exhibiting behavior which would arouse suspicion of rabies infection. Any wild animal that allows you to get close enough to handle it should certainly be suspected of rabies and left alone.

80

Rabies is usually spread when a rabid animal bites another, depositing virus from its saliva into the bite wound. However, rabies virus can enter the body through any break in the skin, through the mucous membranes of the mouth, and probably of the nose and eyes as well. After entering the body, rabies virus becomes "fixed" to nervous tissue where it multiplies. Signs of rabies usually begin between about two weeks and two months following infection, but cases have developed after more than one year from contact.

Rabid cats usually first show changes in their temperament. At this time rabies can be particularly difficult to diagnose because the signs are so variable. A cat may become restless, apprehensive, overly affectionate or shy. A cat will often have a tendency to hide at this stage. Some cats may be febrile (have a fever) and may have dilated pupils. Following these early signs the animal often becomes extremely ferocious, biting or clawing at objects without provocation. This is often referred to as the *furious* form of rabies. These animals become insensible to pain, and, if confined, may bite or slash at the bars of their cages. Partial paralysis of the vocal chords results in a change in their voice. Convulsions may be seen and may cause death.

The *dumb* form of rabies may follow the furious form or may be seen by itself. It is mainly characterized by paralysis. A cat's mouth may hang open and saliva may drip from it. Since such cats cannot ingest food or water they become quite dehydrated. More often, however, cats with the dumb form of rabies develop difficulty walking and then paralysis of the rear legs. Eventually total paralysis occurs, followed by death.

Recovery from rabies is so extremely rare that you might as well not even consider it. Although cats which live completely indoors with no chance of exposure to rabies do not need to be vaccinated, cats which go outdoors, particularly in areas where they may be exposed to rabies carriers, should be vaccinated so you will never have to deal with the problem of owning a rabid animal. Cats should be first vaccinated against rabies when they are three to four months old. There are several types of vaccines available;

81

therefore, the vaccination schedule will have to be determined for your cat individually by your veterinarian. In most cases one or two vaccinations are needed for initial protection followed by booster shots at one or two year intervals.

If you or your cat are exposed to a rabies suspect, that animal should be confined if possible and turned over to a public health officer for rabies quarantine. All bite wounds should be thoroughly washed with large quantities of soap and water. Whether or not your cat will be quarantined following exposure to a rabies suspect will depend on state and local regulations and your cat's vaccination status.

Internal and External Parasites

How To Use This Section Of The Book

Parasites are creatures which are dependent at some point during their life cycle on a host (e.g., your cat). Not all parasites are harmful. In fact, in most well-cared-for small animals, owners overrate them as causes of illness. Certain parasites, under specific circumstances do cause disease; however, don't *assume* that because your cat is sick they have worms or because they're scratching they must have fleas.

If you think your cat has a parasite problem, look for the signs in the Index of Signs (see page 113). (Remember, though, not all animals with parasite infection show signs.) If you find the signs, turn to the appropriate pages and use the information there to help you decide whether or not you need to see a veterinarian. In most cases of internal parasite infection you will need professional help. Many times you can correct an external parasite problem yourself.

If you don't think your cat has a parasite problem, it's a good idea to find time to read or skim this section to complete your knowledge of preventive medicine. I've included the information here in the preventive medicine group because the key to a successful fight against parasites is good prevention and control, which requires good daily care. If you fail to take into account the life cycle of certain parasites in your general daily care, you may continue to

82

have a problem even though you have administered treatment against the parasite on or inside the cat. Learning about the different parasites discussed here will help you provide a healthy environment preventing serious infection and reinfection of your cat and preventing human infection (with certain parasites) as well.

As with the diseases in the Diagnostic Medicine section only the relatively common parasites of cats are discussed here. They are:

Internal parasites—protozoa (page 83), flukes (page 86), tapeworms (page 86), and the following roundworms: ascarids (page 88), hookworms (page 91), stomach worms, (page 92), threadworms (page 92), lungworms (page 92), whipworms (page 93), eyeworms (page 93), heartworms (page 94).

External parasites—fleas (page 95), ticks (page 98), lice (page 99), mites (page 99), flies (page 103).

INTERNAL PARASITES

The *endoparasites* consist of *protozoa, trematodes,* (flukes), *cestodes* (tapeworms) and *nematodes* (roundworms). For the most part, the adults of these parasites live in the intestines. *They can be present with or without causing illness, and you may or may not see them in your cat's stool.* Only if your cat is infected with one of the larger forms *may* you be able to actually see the parasite. If you think your cat has intestinal parasites but can't be sure because you have not seen them, or if you have a new kitten, take a fresh fecal sample to your veterinarian. (A tablespoonful is plenty.) Veterinarians use special procedures to separate the parasites and/or their eggs from the stool and look for evidence of infection microscopically.

A Fecal Sample May Be Important

Protozoa

There are few intestinal protozoa that cause illness in cats. Signs of infection, if present, are variable but often include diarrhea not responsive to home treatment. There is no method to diagnose or treat these parasites successfully at

83

home so you must rely on the help of a veterinarian who can diagnose their presence microscopically and prescribe proper medication.

Toxoplasma Infection   One protozoan of special interest is *Toxoplasma gondii.* This microscopic organism, which is found in all parts of the world, belongs to a class of protozoa known as *coccidia.* Like other members of its class it is able to produce signs of intestinal disease (e.g., diarrhea) in cats, but it also has a tissue phase which can produce serious generalized disease and at times become a human health hazard.

How Toxoplasma Is Acquired   Cats and other mammals, including humans, may acquire *Toxoplasma* infection before birth when infection is

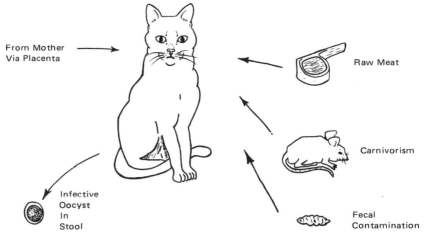

From Mother Via Placenta

Raw Meat

Carnivorism

Infective Oocyst In Stool

Fecal Contamination

acquired by the mother during pregnancy or a previously acquired infection becomes active. More likely sources of infection for a pet cat are the consumption of raw or undercooked meat (including wild caught rodents) containing infective tissue stages of the organism or the ingestion of *Signs Of Toxoplasma* infective *oocysts* which are passed in the feces of certain infected cats. After infection, signs of disease may or may not be seen depending on many factors, including age and general state of health. If signs do develop, they may be as simple as diarrhea or so complex as to mimic many other diseases. Signs which have been seen include fever, lack of appetite, enlarged lymph nodes, weightloss, coughing and difficulty breathing, signs of liver disease including vomiting

84

and yellowish gums, and eye or nervous system problems. Pregnant cats may abort. It is apparent that because of the many possibilities involved, diagnosis must be made by a veterinarian who will use laboratory tests as an aid.

Toxoplasma Infection In Humans Is Not Usually Serious

Alarmist articles concerning toxoplasmosis in people and in cats have appeared in popular magazines. They have often emphasized the congenital type of transmission in pregnant women which can result in severe birth defects and infant death, and they have often dwelt on the possibility of acquiring infection from cat stool. In fact, birth defects due to *Toxoplasma* infection are rare, and the disease in humans is commonly so mild that it passes undiagnosed. Research indicates that five to fifty percent of Americans have had toxoplasmosis; in other countries the incidence is much higher. Although human infection can be acquired from material contaminated with infected cat feces, raw or undercooked meat is to be incriminated in many cases. (Infection rates of greater than eighty percent have been found in people consuming large quantities of raw meat.)

Toxoplasmosis Prevention

Prevent toxoplasmosis in your cat by observing the following rules:

1) Feed commercial cat foods which have been subjected to heat during processing, and cook all meat (heat through to 140° F) you choose to offer to your cat. (Meat frozen to temperatures below -68° F (-20° C) and thawed before feeding is safe, but most home freezers cannot meet these requirements.)

2) Confine your cat to prevent capture and consumption of *Toxoplasma* infected birds or rodents and to prevent contact with the feces of infected carrier animals.

Blood tests are available through your physician if you would like to find out whether you have been infected by *Toxoplasma* and are, therefore, immune to further infection. Pregnant women, in particular, not previously infected should strictly follow the recommendations below for prevention of *Toxoplasma* infection.

1) Avoid eating raw or undercooked meat of any type (heat meat through to 140° F, 60° C), and wash hands after handling raw meat.

85

2) Cats showing otherwise unresponsive signs of illness should be examined by a veterinarian who can perform a fecal examination for *Toxoplasma* organisms. Cats shedding oocysts should be hospitalized or isolated in some other manner until the shedding stops (in about ten to fourteen days) to prevent further transmission of the organism.

3) Follow the rules for preventing *Toxoplasma* infection of cats.

4) Avoid careless handling of stools of cats which are allowed to contact sources of *Toxoplasma* infection. Remove stool from the litter box daily (organisms in stool take two to four days at room temperature to become infective) and use disposable pan liners or disposable cat boxes. Nondisposable cat litter pans should be scalded or disinfected with ten percent ammonia solution. Wear disposable gloves while cleaning the litter pan.

5) Wear gloves while gardening to prevent contact with *Toxoplasma* contaminated soil, and cover children's sandboxes when not in use to prevent fecal contamination.

6) Control cockroaches and flies, rodents and stray cats which can act as transport hosts and carriers of the organism.

Flukes (Trematodes)

Trematode parasites, like protozoa, are uncommon causes of illness in cats. There are several kinds of these flat worms which parasitize different parts of the body of infected animals including the lungs, liver and small intestines. Signs of infection vary greatly and diagnosis must be made by a veterinarian. You can prevent infection of your cat by flukes by restricting hunting since infection is usually acquired by ingesting prey, including raw fish, certain crayfish or crabs, frogs or snails.

Tapeworms (Cestodes)

Cats acquire tapeworms by eating any of three types of infected materials: 1) prey, offal (discarded animal parts) or uncooked meat, 2) raw, fresh water fish, or 3) infected fleas or biting lice. The common tapeworms (*Taenia* sp., *Dypylidium caninum*) are acquired by ingesting prey or

86

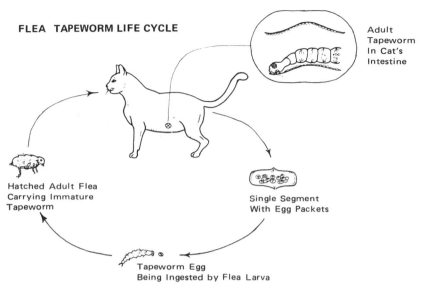

FLEA TAPEWORM LIFE CYCLE

Adult Tapeworm In Cat's Intestine

Hatched Adult Flea Carrying Immature Tapeworm

Single Segment With Egg Packets

Tapeworm Egg Being Ingested by Flea Larva

infected fleas and have similar life cycles:

The adult tapeworm consists of a head with hooks and suckers which attaches to the intestinal wall and a body consisting of a series of reproductive segments. It obtains nourishment by absorbing nutrients in the digestive tract directly through the cuticle which covers each body segment. Eggs produced by the adult tapeworm pass out with the cat's feces and are eaten by an intermediate host (such as a rabbit, rodent, or flea) where they grow into an infective stage commonly called a "bladderworm." When the cat eats an intermediate host, this immature form completes the life cycle by becoming an adult tapeworm in the cat. The life cycle of tapeworms acquired from fish is more complex.

Although heavy tapeworm infestations can cause poor growth or coat changes, variable appetite or gastrointestinal disturbances, in general you will have no reason to suspect infection until you see tapeworm segments clinging to the hair or skin around the anus or in a fresh bowel movement. Fresh tapeworm segments are opaque white or pinkish white, flat and somewhat rectangularly shaped. They often move with a stretching out and shrinking back motion. When dry, the segments become yellow or off-white, translucent and shaped somewhat like grains of rice. Tapeworm segments are

Diagnosing Tapeworms

87

not always present with tapeworm infection. When absent, diagnosis may possibly be made through microscopic fecal examination.

In most cases it is easy to rid a cat of tapeworms. If you demonstrate that your cat has tapeworms, most veterinarians will supply you with safe, tapeworm-killing medication which can be administered at home without unpleasant side effects, such as vomiting or diarrhea. Sometimes, however, the deworming must be done in the veterinary hospital.

Avoid using anti-tapeworm drugs available in pet stores. Most are ineffective. Effective over-the-counter drugs, containing arecoline, cause purgation and can be dangerous. They may cause excessive vomiting, severe diarrhea, and sometimes convulsions and are not recommended for use in cats. After deworming with a product recommended by your veterinarian, make an effort to prevent your cat from re-exposure to sources of tapeworm infection (e.g., flea control is very important). If you don't, deworming may have to be repeated several times a year.

Can people get tapeworms from their cats? In general, the answer is no. Cat tapeworms, unlike some found in dogs, are not human health hazards. In rare instances small children have gotten a tapeworm following accidental ingestion of a flea, but the chance of this occurring is so small that it should be no cause for concern.

Roundworms (Nematodes)

Although most people are aware that roundworm infections occur in cats, most are unaware that, like the other classes of internal parasites, there are several kinds of roundworms. Common ones are covered in the following pages.

Ascarids

Ascarids are the type of roundworms commonly seen in the stool of kittens. They are white, cylindrical and pointed at both ends. They may be relatively small and threadlike in appearance or as long as three or four inches, somewhat resembling small white earthworms. Adult ascarids live in the

88

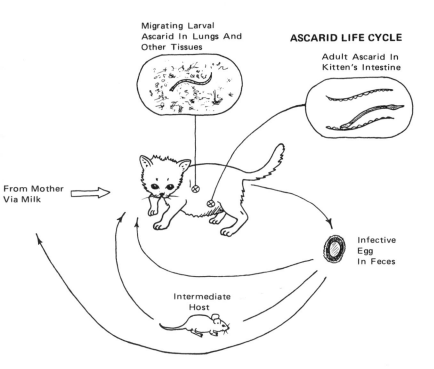

Migrating Larval Ascarid In Lungs And Other Tissues

ASCARID LIFE CYCLE

Adult Ascarid In Kitten's Intestine

From Mother Via Milk

Infective Egg In Feces

Intermediate Host

small intestine and get their nourishment by absorbing nutrients in the digestive juices through their cuticle (outer covering). Mature ascarids produce eggs which pass out in the cat's stool. After about one to four weeks the eggs become infective and contain larval worms. If the infective eggs are ingested by the proper host, they complete their life cycle eventually becoming adult worms in the intestine. If they are eaten by an abnormal host, such as a rodent or cockroach, the larval worms encyst in the tissues of this host where they remain unless a cat or other animal eats the abnormal host and through digestion releases the larvae.

Larvae of the common cat roundworm, *Toxocara cati*, can be transmitted from an adult female cat through the milk to nursing kittens so infection may be found in very young cats. It is impossible to prevent this early infection by deworming the female before she gives birth. Therefore it is probably easiest and best in terms of possible effects on human health to assume that all kittens have ascarid infections and to deworm them routinely.

Ascarid Infection May Occur Soon After Birth

89

Ascarids do not usually cause apparent disease in adult cats. Heavy infections with *Toxocara cati*, in kittens in particular, can, however, lead to death. This roundworm migrates through the lungs en route to the intestine and can cause a cough or even pneumonia. More commonly, vomiting (of worms, sometimes), diarrhea and progressive weakness are seen. Severely infected kittens may have dull coats and pot-bellies on a thin frame.

Salts of the drug *piperazine* are used to remove adult ascarids from the intestines. Piperazine is a very safe and effective drug which you can obtain from your veterinarian or a pet shop and which can be administered at home. There is no need to fast your cat before administering piperazine, and it does not usually cause vomiting or diarrhea. Kittens can be dewormed as early as two or three weeks after birth in order to remove ascarids before they start shedding eggs into the stool, resulting in environmental contamination. Deworming should be repeated *at least* once in two to four weeks to remove any adult worms which were immature and not killed at the first dosing. In extremely heavy infections, deworming may have to be repeated several times before all worms present are killed.

Ascarid eggs are very resistant to environmental stresses. They can remain alive and infective for months once they have contaminated the soil (or litter pan). These factors make it very important to practice good sanitation to prevent reinfection of your own cat, and infection of other cats and possibly humans. Stools should be removed at least weekly (preferably daily) and litter pans should be washed thoroughly with detergents and hot water. Rodents and cockroaches, which may serve as intermediate hosts for the worms, should be controlled.

Although feline ascarids do not occur in human intestines, their larvae *may* cause *viseral larval migrans*, a rare condition in which roundworm larvae migrate in the body. *Viseral larval migrans* may cause anything from no signs of illness to severe signs, including blindness. It occurs most often in young children who play in soil infested with the eggs of the common *dog* roundworm, *Toxocara canis*, and put their contaminated hands in their mouths. But *Toxocara cati* has been incriminated in some cases. Although complete recovery is the rule, the possibility of human infection is a significant reason for good ascarid control and for good general hygiene.

Hookworms

Hookworms are small intestinal parasites (about one-fourth to one-half inch long) which attach to the wall of the small intestine and suck blood. Cats may become infected by ingesting infective larval worms off the ground or by penetration of the skin by infective larvae. Kittens may become infected before birth by larvae migrating in the mother's body tissues and shortly after birth via larvae passed in colostrum.

Migration of hookworm larvae through the skin can cause itching reflected by scratching, redness and sometimes bumps and scabs on the skin. Hookworms living in the intestine can cause diarrhea, severe anemia, weakness, and emaciation leading to death. Infection in young animals sometimes causes anemia and death even before hookworm eggs are detectable in the stool.

Hookworms cannot be diagnosed and treated effectively without the aid of a veterinarian. Hookworms are small enough to be overlooked even when they are passed in the stool. Signs of illness caused by hookworm infection can be caused by other diseases as well. The safest and most effective compounds for treatment are available only through veterinarians. If your cat has to be treated for hookworms, your veterinarian will probably use a drug called *disophenol* and keep your cat in the hospital, or a compound called *dichlorvos* which you may or may not be able to administer at home. Other kinds of safe, effective drugs may soon be available as well.

Hookworms are a problem only in areas which provide an environment suitable for the development of infective larvae. The pre-infective stages require moderate temperatures (between about seventy-three and eighty-six degrees F) and moisture for development. Prevent re-infection or spread

Possible Signs Of Hookworms

Diagnosis And Treatment

How To Prevent Hookworm Infection

91

of hookworms by keeping your cat indoors and having them use a litter pan which is thoroughly cleaned *at least* weekly (preferably daily) until your cat is diagnosed as hookworm free. Cage areas should be washed daily and allowed to dry, and outdoor areas where stool may have been deposited must be kept dry for three weeks to kill larvae.

Stomach Worms

Stomach worms infect both cats and dogs and occur mainly in the southeastern United States. They cause frequent vomiting which cannot be differentiated from other causes of vomiting without an examination of a fecal sample and the aid of a veterinarian. You can prevent infection of your cat by preventing the ingestion of cockroaches, crickets, and beetles which serve as intermediate hosts for the development of the worm. (In heavily infested areas this would mean you will probably have to keep cats indoors or supervise them outdoors to prevent hunting.) Piperazine salts (e.g., piperazine adipate, piperazine citrate) are used for treatment.

Threadworms

The threadworm, *Strongyloides stercoralis*, is a round-worm parasite of cats, dogs, and man. Infection is acquired most commonly when infective larvae penetrate the skin. This can cause red lumps, crusts and scratching. And during their migration through the body the larvae can produce signs of respiratory disease, such as a cough. Cats can also become infected by ingestion of infective larvae. Threadworms are very small worms and will not be seen in the stool. When diagnosis is established by a veterinarian, a drug called thiabendazole is often used for treatment. Prevent *Strongyloides* infection by providing your cat with a clean, dry environment.

Lungworms

Lungworms, as their name implies, are small (about one-fourth inch long) roundworms who as adults live in the lungs of cats. The more common lungworm, *Aleurostron-*

gylus abstrussus, infects cats who have eaten snails, slugs, rodents, frogs, lizards or birds carrying infective larvae of the worm. These intermediate and transfer hosts become infected when they ingest larvae which have been coughed up and passed in the stool of affected cats. Although infection is uncommon, lungworms do occur in many areas all over the United States and Europe so an informed cat owner should be aware of their occurrence.

The first sign of lungworm infection is usually a persistant cough, often accompanied by a gradual weight loss. Other signs in addition to cough can be fever, loss of appetite, nasal discharge and sneezing. Therefore, it is easy to confuse this disease with other causes of respiratory distress.

Diagnosis and treatment of lungworm disease must be done by a veterinarian since both may be difficult. Veterinarians look for lungworm larvae (or eggs in certain cases) in the stool (or sputum) of infected cats, so it can be helpful to bring a stool sample when you take your cat to be examined. Prevent infection with the common lungworm by restricting your cat's hunting.

Whipworms

Whipworms are intestinal round worms which are known to occur in the dog's *cecum* (part of the large intestine) and sometimes cause diarrhea and weight loss. Although once thought not to occur in cats, whipworms are now being diagnosed in them. Infection is acquired directly by ingesting infective larvae from contaminated soil. Diagnosis must usually be made by a veterinarian since infection is often symptomless. Ask your veterinarian if you live in an area where whipworms are found. If you do, consider having a stool sample examined semi-annually for evidence of whipworm infection.

Eyeworms

Eyeworms are small roundworms (less than one-half inch long) which live in the conjunctival sac of the infected cat. They cause reddening and irritation of the conjunctiva, discharge from the eye and, sometimes, damage to the eyeball itself. They occur on the West Coast of the United

States and are transmitted through the mouthparts of flies which feed on secretions from the eye. You can treat these worms if you find them by removing them with a pair of fine forceps or tweezers.

Heartworms

Heartworms *(Dirofilaria imitis)* are roundworm parasites ranging from six to twelve inches long which occur in the hearts, pulmonary arteries and vena cavae of infected *dogs.* They can cause serious and life threatening disease in dogs and have recently become documented as able to do the same in cats, although rarely. These worms are transmitted by mosquitoes which feed off of infected dogs, and although there are areas where heartworm infection is likely to occur all over the United States, infection in dogs is particularly common along the Atlantic and Gulf Coasts. If your cat spends a great deal of time outdoors and if you live in an endemic area, be sure your veterinarian keeps you informed about the latest developments concerning heartworms in cats.

Pinworms

In answer to a common question: cats, like dogs, do not get or spread pinworms. The human pinworm, *Enterobius vermicularis,* occurs only in humans and higher primates such as chimpanzees.

Trichinosis

Trichinosis is a roundworm infection which occurs when larval forms of *Trichinella spiralis*, which encysts in muscle tissue, are eaten. This disease affects humans, pigs and other mammals including cats and rats. Vomiting, diarrhea (bloody), and signs of muscle involvement including stiffness and weakness, and signs of pain have occurred in affected cats. Although cats are among the animals most susceptible to trichinosis, infection is not frequently recognized. Prevent trichinosis by not feeding raw or undercooked pork and by restricting hunting (to prevent preying on possibly infected rodents).

EXTERNAL PARASITES

External parasites of cats are *arthropods* (hard-coated insects and insect-like animals) which live on cat skin feeding off of blood, tissue fluid or the skin itself.

Fleas

Fleas are probably the most prevalent external parasite of cats. They are wingless, dark brown insects capable of jumping great distances relative to their body size. They obtain nourishment by sucking blood. Fleas are not very host specific; therefore, in spite of the fact that there are several flea species, cat fleas are found on dogs, dog fleas are found on cats, and cat and dog fleas will feed from humans. The important thing is not the kind of flea present, but that a cat should not have fleas. Heavy flea infestation is not a normal and natural condition, and just a few fleas can sometimes be responsible for serious disease. Large numbers of fleas can be responsible for significant loss of blood in kittens, old animals or any weakened cat. This blood loss *(anemia)* can result in death, particularly in young kittens. Fleas are carriers of disease (e.g., tapeworms, see page 86). Allergic dermatitis is also commonly caused by fleas (see page 122).

Female fleas usually lay their eggs off the host. They may lay them on the host, but because the eggs aren't stickly, they usually drop off. Flea eggs are white and about the size of a small grain of salt. If a cat is heavily infested with fleas, eggs may be

ADULT FLEA FEEDING ON CAT

Actual Size

Pupa

Larva
Feeding on Debris

Eggs
In Carpet

95

found in its coat mixed with flea feces (partially digested blood) which are about the same size but colored black. (If moistened with water these black granules will dissolve to produce a blood colored fluid.) The eggs hatch into larvae anywhere from about two days to two weeks after laying. Mature flea larvae resemble very small fly maggots. They are about one-fourth inch long and white to creamy yellow in color. They are usually found in cracks in floors, under carpets, in bedding and in other similar places. The larvae feed only a little, then spin cocoons in which they develop to adult fleas. Larvae may take from ten days to several months to become adult fleas, depending on environmental conditions. Unfed adult fleas can live for several months.

Since a major part of the flea life cycle is off the cat, flea control on a single host is not sufficient to get rid of fleas completely. Flea control must be practiced on all pets living in a house and fleas must be removed from the premises. Washing or burning infected bedding and thorough vacuuming are often sufficient to get rid of small numbers of fleas. In other cases houses or cage areas must be sprayed or fumigated with commercial insecticides or the services of a professional exterminator must be obtained.

If your cat has fleas, the first thing to do, if possible, is to give the cat a good bath. You can use a regular gentle shampoo or a commercial *cat* shampoo containing insecticide to kill fleas. If you use a regular shampoo, remember that you are removing fleas mechanically only. If you don't rinse your cat's coat well, fleas stunned by the water will wake up as the coat drys and still be around to cause trouble. Once your cat is clean, use any of the methods covered below for continued flea control. However, be *sure* that any insecticidal product you choose is marked clearly for use around cats. Cats are very susceptible to the toxic effects of certain chemicals, so products not specifically recommended for use with cats should be avoided.

1) Flea dips are insecticides which are applied to the cat's coat as a liquid and allowed to dry. I think it is easiest to sponge on a dip while the cat is still wet following a bath. Be sure to follow the directions on the package, and be sure

the dip you choose is designed for cats. Sheep dip or dog dips are often toxic to cats as well as irritating to their skin.

Flea Spray Or Powders

2) Flea sprays and powders contain a large variety of insecticides. Fleas may become resistant to certain insecticides, so the most effective powder or spray (or dip) against fleas may change with time. You may want to ask your veterinarian what they currently recommend. Follow package directions carefully, and avoid applying powders or sprays to irritated or raw skin to prevent further irritation.

Flea Collar Or Tag

3) The most effective flea collars contain organophosphate insecticides (e.g., *dichlorvos, naled*) incorporated into a plastic base which allows their slow release. Flea tags also contain insecticide enclosed in a plastic cover to prevent its contact with the skin. Organophosphate chemicals act directly on the parasite causing death. Their action in flea collars is *not* due to absorption by the cat and ingestion by the parasite with a blood meal. In the concentrations found in flea collars and tags for cats, the insecticides used have been found to be quite safe. Flea collars can be used safely on *healthy* cats as young as two months of age, but package directions to the contrary should be heeded. Flea collars should be applied loosely (one or two finger widths between neck and collar) and wetting should be avoided to prevent premature loss of anti-flea effect. Other insecticides should not be applied in the presence of a flea collar or tag unless advised by a veterinarian.

A few cats are sensitive to organophosphates and develop *contact dermatitis* when a flea collar is applied. The dermatitis often first appears as some hair loss and reddening of the neck skin under the collar. If the collar is removed at this time, the condition usually clears up with no other treatment. If the collar is not removed, the skin condition can progress to large raw areas, sometimes secondarily infected with bacteria, which can be difficult to clear up and can need the attention of a veterinarian. Flea collar dermatitis can sometimes be prevented by airing the collar two or three days before putting it on the cat. Cats that cannot wear flea collars often can wear flea tags, which were developed to prevent contact of the insecticides with the

Flea Collars Can Cause Contact Dermatitis

skin.

Flea Stick
4) Flea sticks contain a form of insecticide, *methyl-carbamate,* in a waxy base which allows it to be applied directly to the skin. As with other products for flea control, follow package directions carefully.

Manual Removal
5) Removal of fleas by hand or with a flea comb are extremely ineffective methods of flea control. Of course, if you see a flea, you can try to remove it, but don't rely on this as a means of routine control if other methods can be used.

Home Remedies
6) I have been unable to find substantiation of the effectiveness against fleas of such home remedies as eucalyptus buds and feeding brewer's yeast (B vitamins). If you want to stick to such remedies, examine your cat *thoroughly* for evidence of fleas frequently. And if any are present, re-evaluate your means of flea control.

Sticktight Fleas
The sticktight flea, *Echinophaga gallinacea,* is mainly a parasite of poultry, but can attack cats. You can recognize sticktight fleas easily because the adults stick tight to the cat's skin and don't run off when approached. They are blood suckers and, if found, should be removed manually by the use of a cat flea dip.

Ticks

Ticks are not commonly found on cats, probably because they habitually groom themselves thoroughly. If you live in a woodsy or rural area and your cat goes outside, you may occasionally find a tick. Adult female ticks look different before and after they have taken a blood meal (see illustration); male

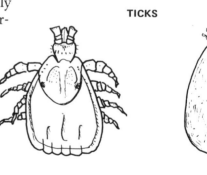

TICKS

Actual Size

Empty

Engor

98

ticks don't swell with feeding. The most serious things ticks usually do is cause an area of skin inflammation at the site of attachment, but their presence should never be ignored.

Since cats rarely have more than one or two ticks on their bodies, the easiest way to remove them is by hand. Using your thumb and first finger, grasp the tick as close as possible to where its mouth parts insert into the cat's skin. Then exert a firm but gentle, constant pull. (There's no need to twist.) If you've pulled just right and gotten the tick at the optimum time after attachment, the whole tick will detach. If the mouth parts are left embedded, don't worry. The tick never grows back, and only rarely does a tick bite become infected. The site of the tick bite usually becomes red and thickened in reaction to a substance secreted in the tick's saliva, but it usually heals in about two weeks. DO NOT try to burn off ticks with a match or apply kerosene, gasoline, or other similar petroleum products. If you feel you must apply something to the tick, use a small amount of concentrated flea or tick dip, alcohol, ether, or acetone (fingernail polish remover), and apply it only to the tick, not to the surrounding skin or hair.

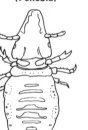

LOUSE
(Felicola)

Actual Size

Lice

Lice are much less commonly seen than fleas or ticks on well-cared-for cats. Adult lice are pale colored and about one-tenth inch or less in length. They spend their entire life on one host, and attach their tiny white eggs to the hair. Some lice require blood or body fluids to live; others eat skin scales. They can cause signs of itching and can carry certain tapeworm larvae. Kill lice with a thorough bath followed by a spray or dip for cats effective against ticks and fleas.

Mites (Mange)

Mange is a general term for infestation with mites. It is not any one single disease in itself. The mites discussed here

99

are ear mites, head mites, and trombiculid mites. Other mite infestations of cats are rare.

Ear Mites

How To Diagnose Ear Mites

Ear mites, *Otodectes cynotis*, live in the ear canal of dogs and cats and feed on skin debris. They cause the formation of large amounts of dark black to reddish brown wax in the ear and usually vigorous ear scratching. An infected cat may hold its ears in an abnormally flattened manner and may shake its head.

If you think your cat has ear mites, remove some of the discharge from the ear canal with a cotton swab. You may be able to see the mites by examining the waxy material in a bright light or by putting it on a piece of black paper. (A magnifying glass may help you.) Live ear mites look like moving white specks about the size of the point of a dressmaker's pin.

Treatment Of Ear Mites

If you have seen mites and there is not much waxy discharge, you may be able to treat the condition at home. DO NOT attempt home treatment unless you have seen the mites. Other ear problems can cause similar discharges and may be complicated by the use of an ear mite preparation. Treatment consists of cleaning out the ears and instilling insecticidal liquid with an eyedropper or dropper bottle. How often this must be done depends on the product used. Whether or not you will need to see a veterinarian to obtain an effective ear mite preparation depends on the area in which you live. Effective preparations often contain one or more of the following ingredients: *pyrethrins, piperonyl butoxide, dichlorophene, rotenone, methoxychlor, lindane.* Again be sure any preparation you choose is safe for cats. If your cat's ears are very dirty or very inflamed, it is best to have them thoroughly cleaned by a veterinarian before treatment is begun.

Head Mites

Head mites, *Notoedres cati*, are microscopic mites which infest cats and which can transiently infest human beings and dogs. These mites burrow beneath the horny layers of the skin causing intense signs of itching followed by hair loss. Because these mites seem to prefer the skin of the head and ears, thickened, wrinkled skin and gray crusts and scales are usually first seen in these areas and on the back of the neck. In neglected cases lesions of this appearance may be found on the feet and under the tail. *Notoedres* infestation is easily spread from cat to cat. *Signs Of Head Mange*

If you suspect that your cat has head mange, infection can only be confirmed by microscopic examination of a skin scraping. Therefore it is advisable to have your cat examined by a veterinarian before beginning treatment for the mites. Not only can they confirm the presence of mites and give you detailed information on the use of a proper insecticide to prevent toxicity to your cat, but a veterinarian can also administer a *corticosteroid* (see page 212), if necessary, to help relieve the itching until the mites are completely gone, and antibiotics in cases of secondary bacterial infection. *Diagnosis Of Head Mange*

If you cannot obtain the services of a veterinarian and choose to begin treatment yourself, be sure to pick an insecticide marked clearly as safe for cats and follow the directions on it carefully. Treatment consists of clipping affected areas on long-haired cats and applying sulfur or rotenone preparations, or bathing and applying a dip which kills *Notoedres* twice at seven to ten day intervals. Dips effective against *Notoedres* and reported safe for cats include 2.5% dilution of lime sulfur (orchard spray available at garden stores), and 0.2% malathion. *Home Treatment Is Possible*

Trombiculid Mites (Chiggers)

Trombiculid mites (chiggers, harvest mites) are red, orange or yellowish mites which have larvae that are parasitic

101

on cats and other mammals. (The nymphs and adults feed on plants or invertebrates.) The larvae are often found on the head and neck, particularly in and around the ears, but can infest any part of the body, causing scratching which is sometimes very severe. Look for red, orange, or yellowish specks about the size of the point of a dressmaker's pin in affected areas. Use a magnifying glass, if necessary. If you

Parasites Shared By Cats and Dogs		
Cat		**Dog**

External Parasites

Fleas	⟶ ⟵	Fleas
Ear Mites	⟶ ⟵	Ear Mites

Internal Parasites

Protozoa: Coccidia	via environmental contamination with stool ⟶ ⟵	Protozoa: Coccidia
Toxoplasma	via environmental contamination with stool ⟶	*Toxoplasma*
Tapeworms *(Dypylidium)*	via ingested fleas ⟶ ⟵	Tapeworms *(Dypylidium)*
Ascarids *(Toxascaris leonina* only)	via environmental contamination with stool ⟶ ⟵	Ascarids *(Toxascaris leonina* only)
Threadworms	via environmental contamination with stool ⟶ ⟵	Threadworms
Hookworms	via environmental contamination with stool ⟶ ⟵	Hookworms
Stomach Worms	via ingested beetles, etc. ⟶ ⟵	Stomach Worms

cannot find the mites, diagnosis may have to be made with a skin scraping performed by a veterinarian. Mites found solely in the ear can be eliminated by the treatments for ear mites (see page 100). Mites in other areas can be controlled with dips or other preparations effective against head mites.

Flies
Adult flies are not normally parasitic on cats. Some types of adult flies lay their eggs in raw or infected wounds. When the eggs hatch, the maggots feed on the tissue present, producing a condition called *myasis*. I've frequently seen maggots in infected ears as well as in neglected skin wounds and under matted hair. To treat myasis, all the maggots must be removed manually, the areas washed with an antibacterial soap (e.g., Phisohex®), and a topical antibiotic cream or ointment applied to treat any secondary bacterial infection which may be present. It is extremely important to treat the predisposing condition or myasis is likely to recur.

Value of Preventive Medicine
Begin to practice these preventive medicine techniques as soon as you take a new cat into your home. In a short time the proper way to care for a healthy cat will become second nature to you. The effects of poor preventive techniques early in a cat's life can sometimes never be reversed. On the other hand, a cat that is fed well, groomed regularly and kept in a clean and parasite-free environment will have a good start on a long and healthy life. Combine these things with love and proper training and a yearly visit to a veterinarian for booster shots and examination, and you should find that living with your cat is a simple, enjoyable and rewarding experience.

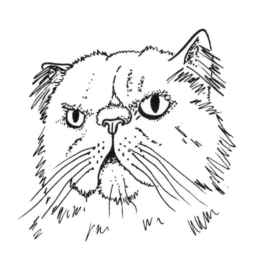

Diagnostic Medicine —
What to do When Your Cat is Sick

Diagnostic Medicine

General Procedure for Diagnosing Signs

If you have been giving your cat the kind of good care you have learned about in the first part of this book, but illness occurs, you are not necessarily at fault. Even the most well-cared-for cat may become sick or injured. The following pages on diagnostic medicine and the sections on emergency medicine and geriatric medicine are here to help you in such situations. The best way to use these three sections, as with the rest of the book, is to read them through completely and become familiar with the contents. In this way, when a problem occurs you will not have to "waste" time in an attempt to digest the new material. You will already know how to deal with the problem or a quick review will be all that is necessary. Knowing the contents ahead of time will also help you to prevent certain problems, for example, *wound infection* page 118 and *poisoning* page 176. Another way (that you will want to use if your cat is already sick) is to use the index to signs of illness and the general index for the book.

The *Index of Signs* is an alphabetical listing of the changes which may occur when your cat is sick. *Symptoms* are subjective indicators of disease. Because your cat cannot describe their feelings in words, they technically have no symptoms, only *signs*, which are any objective evidence of disease or injury you can detect. To use the *Index of Signs*, first determine what your cat's signs are. For example: you *see* scratching (not itching, your cat *feels* itching) and you

107

feel scabs and bumps on your cat's skin. Then look up these changes in the *Index of Signs* and turn to the pages listed there to find out about the problem and what to do for a cure. If you can't find the signs you see or can't put the signs into words, look in the *General Index* under the body part that is involved, for example: *Skin.* Also use the General Index whenever you want to read about a general subject (e.g., breeding) or a particular disease (e.g., rabies). Signs are included in the *General Index* in addition to their presence in the *Index of Signs.* Remember only relatively common problems are discussed here in terms of home treatment. If you don't find what you are looking for in either index, consult a veterinarian. The problem may or may not be serious, but is not one I've found "run of the mill" for the general cat population.

You should watch carefully for signs of illness. Sometimes a cat is very sick before signs of illness are obvious (even to a practiced eye). Because cats can't talk, the practice of veterinary medicine is often more difficult than that of human medicine. Since you are closest to your cat, you may be able to notice signs of illness before your veterinarian can find any abnormalities on a simple physical examination. Anything you can tell your veterinarian in the way of signs may be *very* important.

Relatively few signs signal the presence of many diseases. Very different diseases often cause the same signs and sometimes can only be differentiated from one another by specialized diagnostic aids, such as x-rays and blood tests. Keep this in mind if you think your cat has all the signs of a particular illness but fails to respond to the suggested treatment. Keep in mind also the value of *intuition* in recognizing that your cat is ill or injured. You are closest to your cat. If "something just doesn't seem right," sit down with your cat, take their temperature (see page 194) and perform a physical examination (see *Anatomy* page 9). Often you will turn up specific signs which you can read about and deal with at home. If you don't, don't assume that you are wrong and that your cat is O.K. Rely on your intuition and get your cat examined by a veterinarian. They

108

may find something you missed and can perform specialized tests if necessary.

Three common general signs of illness which accompany many illnesses are *change in behavior, change in appetite,* and *fever.* Two other signs you may often see are *dehydration* and *shivering.*

Don't take any change of behavior lightly. One of the first signs in most cat illnesses is a change in behavior in which the cat becomes more quiet and less active (*depression* of activity). Any time this occurs it should alert you to at least take your cat's temperature, and if the sign persists, perform a complete physical examination or obtain the services of a veterinarian. Although most cats become less active and more quiet when they are sick or injured, any behavioral change can indicate a medical problem. Cats can have "emotional" (behavioral) problems as well, but expert advice is needed to correct such problems, and this book is not designed to help you solve them. *[Change Of Behavior]*

Cats frequently lose their appetites completely when they are sick *(anorexia).* Often, however, you will notice only a *change* in appetite. The sick cat may eat less or more. And, although one day's change is not usually important, it should alert you to look for a possible health problem. Once a cat is grown, its appetite and activities are fairly constant from day to day. Changes which persist longer than five days with no other signs of illness should be discussed with your veterinarian. Changes in appetite accompanied by other signs should not be allowed to continue longer than twenty-four hours before you or your veterinarian investigates the problem. *[Change Of Appetite]*

The normal resting cat usually maintains its rectal temperature within the range of 101.0 to 102.5 degrees F. (For how to take a cat's temperature see page 194). An elevated body temperature *(fever)* usually indicates infection (most often bacterial or viral in nature), but keep in mind that factors such as exercise, excitement and high environmental temperature can elevate a cat's temperature as well. Many kinds of bacteria produce toxins which cause the body to release chemical substances called *pyrogens* that *[Fever]* produce fever. The way other agents produce fever is not known, but is probably also related to the body's release of pyrogens.

It is important to remember that fever is a sign of disease, not a disease in itself. Although drugs can be used to lower an extremely high fever (greater than 106° F), the most common drug used for this purpose, aspirin, must be used with extreme caution in cats. The important thing is to find the cause of the fever and treat that, not the fever itself. In fact, there are indications that the presence of fever may even be beneficial in some diseases.

Except in kittens less than four weeks old, lowered body temperature (less than 100° F) is usually indicative of overwhelming disease and the affected animal needs immediate care.

Dehydration   All body tissues are bathed in tissue fluids consisting primarily of water, ions, protein and some other chemical substances such as nutrients and waste products. Normal tissue fluids are extremely important in maintaining normal cellular functions. Changes in the body's water composition are always accompanied by changes in other constituents of tissue fluids. Small changes can have important consequences.

The most common tissue fluid alteration seen in sick animals is depletion of body water – *dehydration*. Dehydration occurs whenever the body's output of water exceeds its intake. One common cause of dehydration during illness is the failure of water intake sufficient to meet the body's fixed daily requirements. Water is continually lost in urine, feces, with respiratory gases, and by evaporation from some body surfaces (minor in cats). Since cats frequently stop eating and often drink little when sick, their basic daily needs are not met and dehydration easily occurs. Dehydration also occurs in conditions which cause excessive water and/or *electrolyte* (ion) loss, such as vomiting and diarrhea. In addition, the presence of fever increases the body's water needs.

Although dehydration begins as soon as water output exceeds intake, the signs of dehydration are usually undetectable until a water deficit of about four percent of

110

total body weight has been incurred. If your cat has visible signs of dehydration, they may have been sick longer than you realize and need professional veterinary care.

1) *Decreased elasticity of skin.* The tissues beneath the skin contain a large portion of the total body water. Because this water compartment is one of the least important to the ·body, it is drawn upon first in a situation of dehydration. To test for dehydration, pick up a fold of skin along the middle of the back and let it drop. In a well-hydrated, normally-fleshed cat the skin springs immediately back into place. In a moderately dehydrated cat the skin moves slowly into place. In severe dehydration the skin may form a tent. (Fat animals tend to have more elastic skin than thin ones.)

Signs Of Dehydration (According To Increasing Severity)

2) *Dryness of the mucous membranes lining the mouth and eyes.* This may be difficult to evaluate until dehydration becomes severe.

3) *Sunken eyes.* This condition can also be due to severe weight loss, but in any case it's serious.

4) *Circulatory collapse (shock).* See *Emergency Medicine* page 169. Mild dehydration and its accompanying ion imbalance can be prevented and/or corrected by administering water and nutrients orally. In more severe dehydration, or with diseases which prevent oral intake, fluids must be administered by other routes. In such cases veterinarians administer fluids *subcutaneously* (under the skin) or *intravenously* (directly into the bloodstream), if necessary. Fluids given via these routes are sterile and of varied composition. The fluid your veterinarian chooses will depend on the route of administration and the cause of dehydration. Good fluid therapy is an important part of the care of almost all animals sick enough to require hospitalization.

Shivering may or may not be a sign of illness. Many cats shiver when frightened, excited or emotionally upset. In fact, this is the most common type of shivering. Cats may also shiver when they are cold. Like people, unless they are accustomed to being outside in cool weather without protection, cats get cold and shiver in an attempt to increase body heat.

Shivering

Shivering may also be a sign of pain. When associated

111

with pain it often accompanies the kind of pain that is difficult to localize, such as abdominal or spinal pain. Another time shivering is associated with illness is during the early part of a febrile disease (illness with fever). The heat shivering produces contributes to the rising temperature.

If your cat is shivering, try to eliminate emotional causes and take their temperature before concluding that this sign is due to pain.

When you determine the signs your cat has and have read about their condition, you will need to begin treatment. If you do not already know how to proceed with the treatment involved or need more information on the care of a sick cat, see the section on nursing at home, page 193.

Times When A Veterinarian's Help Is Needed

Any emergency.

Whenever you fail to diagnose the problem.

Whenever home treatment fails.

For any problem which requires x-ray pictures, laboratory analysis, or anesthesia.

For any problem requiring prescription drugs, including antibiotics.

For yearly physical examination and booster vaccination.

Index of Signs

114

S **Scabs,** on body skin 91, 92, 122, 124 (see also Scratching)
on ears 100, 101, 132

Scooting on anus 153

Scratching, at body skin 91, 92, 99, 101, 102, 122, 123
at ears 100, 102, 132

Sexual attractiveness 220

"Shh" sound in heart beat 163, 189

Shivering 111, 177, 183

Shock 168, 177

Smell, abnormal
at anus 20 (see also Diarrhea)
at vulva 239
from ears 132
from mouth 134, 188
on body skin 120

Sneezing 93, 135, 136, 138

Squinting 93, 128, 130

Stool, dark-colored 30, 69
in house 50, 150
loose (see Diarrhea)
loss of control of 163, 175

Straining, to defecate 152
to urinate 156, 157

Sunken eyes 111

Swallowing, difficult 81, 133, 172

Swelling, at anus 120, 153
inside ear 120, 132, 133
of breast 126
of foot or limb 120, 143, 145
of lumps nodes 30, 84, 165
of vulva 220
of wound 119
on face 120, 125, 180
under skin 119, 120, 125, 143, 180

T **Tearing,** excessive 93, 128, 129, 130, 135

Teeth, discolored 56, 134
extra 29
loose 28, 58
missing 28

Testes, undescended 32, 227

Thickened skin, on body 101, 122, 125

Skin

In addition to the information in this section, other causes of skin disease will be found in the sections on external parasites (see page 95) and nutrition (see page 58).

Wounds, Wound Infection and Abscesses

Wounds and their frequent sequelae *abscesses* are the most common skin problems seen in cats that are allowed outdoors. Whether or not your cat needs to see a veterinarian following a wound depends a lot on the kind of wound it is. Short, clean *lacerations* (cuts) or cuts which do not completely penetrate the skin and most *abrasions* (scrapes) usually need only to be washed thoroughly with mild soap and rinsed with large volumes of warm, clean water. After thorough washing they should be examined daily for signs of infection. Larger cuts (about one-half inch long or longer) and punctures usually need veterinary attention.

How Wounds Heal   Wound healing is essentially the same process whether it occurs by *primary* or *secondary* intention. The wound fills with a clot. The wound edges contract, reducing the wound in size. White blood cells called *macrophages* enter the wound and remove dead tissue and foreign material. Blood vessels and connective tissue cells enter the wound followed by nerve fibers and lymphatic cells. At the same time this is happening, skin cells move in to close the surface defect, and finally the wound is healed. Wounds which are allowed to heal without apposing (bringing together) their edges heal by *secondary intention.* Healing by *primary intention* is more rapid. Your veterinarian tries to achieve primary intention healing by suturing larger wounds closed. Suturing clean wounds closed also helps prevent them from becoming infected while they are healing. Wounds, however, which are likely to become infected cannot be sutured closed or must be sutured only with special care. Puncture type wounds, most commonly bite wounds or claw wounds, are among the most frequently seen wounds on cats which fall into this category.

118

Bite wounds and claw wounds require special attention not only because they are likely to become infected (which interferes with healing), but also because if the body's defenses (white blood cells and lymph nodes) are unable to overcome the bacteria, infection may spread from the original wound to the blood stream. They may result in a *septicemia* (bacterial toxins in the blood) or a *bacteremia* (actual bacteria in the blood) and can sometimes eventually lead to death. Although puncture type wounds are difficult to wash, you should make an attempt to clean them thoroughly whenever you notice them on your cat. Flushing three percent *hydrogen peroxide* into the wound under pressure (bulb syringe, eye dropper) is one of the best home remedies because its foaming action tends to wash debris from the wound. If possible, antibiotics should be administered by a veterinarian at the start of treatment (within twenty-four hours of the wound's incurrence) since this type of wound is so prone to infection. If you choose to treat the wound only with home care, you can try instilling over-the-counter antibiotic ointments into the wound to help prevent infection, but be sure to take your cat's temperature daily and examine the wound carefully each time you do for local signs of infection. (For more on how to clean and treat a puncture wound, see page 121.)

Most wounds show signs of *inflammation* — a small area of reddening around the wound (not prominent in cats), slight swelling, warmth and possibly pain — but these signs usually disappear within forty-eight hours if infection is not present. If the swelling, redness, warmth and pain remain or are getting worse or if you see unhealthy looking tissue or pus-like fluid draining from the wound, infection is probably present and examination by a veterinarian may be necessary. Fever, whether or not accompanied by local signs of wound infection, requires examination by a veterinarian who can administer appropriate antibiotics.

An *abscess* is a localized collection of pus in a cavity caused by the death and

Scab

Pus

119

destruction of body tissues. Abscesses are the most common type of infection established following improperly treated bite or claw wounds. They usually cause swelling under the skin at the wound site and sometimes signs of pain, but often go unnoticed until they begin to drain sticky white, yellow to yellow-green or blood-tinged pus. Abscesses are frequently found on the head (cheeks, ears), legs and feet, and on the tail (near its base). Much less frequently they occur in the tissues behind the eye causing swelling, protrusion of the eye and signs of pain particularly when attempts are made to open the mouth. Veterinarians treat abscesses by opening them surgically under anesthesia and by removing all visibly dead and infected tissue *(debridement)*. Antibiotics are administered and you are usually instructed to clean the wound daily at home. You can often tell when an abscess which is not draining is formed and ready to open by feeling it with your finger. If you can feel a soft spot or the swelling feels fluid filled under the skin, it is ready to lance. Sometimes your veterinarian will advise you to put warm packs on an inflamed and infected area which is not yet abscessed. This helps localize the infection so effective drainage can be provided. By transiently increasing the blood supply to the area, hot packs may help antibiotics get into the infection preventing abscessation in some instances. You may want to try this without a veterinarian's advice on an infected diffuse swelling *(cellulitis)* which has not yet abscessed if your cat does not have a fever and seems fairly normal except for the signs of inflammation.

Home Treatment For Abscesses   If your cat has a well-localized abscess which has burst or is covered by a scab which can be removed and has *no fever,* you may be able to get the abscess to heal with home treatment alone. You must pull off the scab if the abscess is not yet draining, then determine how extensive the abscess is. Any abscess in which you can't reach to the full extent of the pocket probably won't heal but spread or recur and needs a veterinarian's attention. Determine the extent of the pocket by wrapping your finger in a sterile gauze pad and probing the wound thoroughly. Be gentle, but be sure to clean out all pus and loose tissue and to probe to the wound's farthest

120

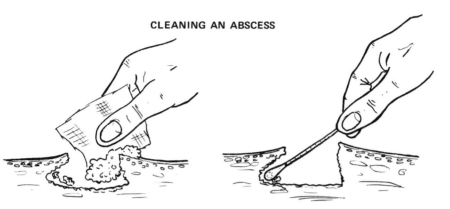

reaches. A small abscess can be cleaned and probed with a cotton-tipped swab. Flush the open abscess thoroughly with hydrogen peroxide once or twice a day.

Hydrogen peroxide is an unstable solution which decomposes to water and oxygen when it comes into contact with tissue. When it decomposes it has a transient and weak germicidal effect, and it forms bubbles which are effective in removing debris from infected wounds. If the opening of the wound is large enough, you can pour the solution directly into it. A syringe (bulb or hypodermic type) or eye dropper can be used to flush the solution into smaller wounds. The hydrogen peroxide can be applied to a gauze pad which is used to wipe the wound or to a cotton-tipped swab which can be inserted into very small wounds. As the solution bubbles, it becomes warm. Some cats find this very uncomfortable. Clean the wound until visible tissue is free of debris and/or until the solution runs clear. Repeat the cleaning once or twice a day until debris no longer accumulates in the wound.

If your cat has a fever or any other signs of illness accompanying an abscess or wound, DO NOT attempt home treatment without the help of a veterinarian. Fever and/or other general signs of illness indicate that the problem is a more serious infection which the body's defenses have not been able to localize. Improperly treated wounds can be responsible for serious and expensive complications — among them bone infections, recurrent abscesses, and bacterial

Times To Seek Veterinary Help With Abscesses

121

infections of internal organs such as the liver, heart and lungs.

Allergic Dermatitis

Some cats, like some people, are born with the predisposition to develop reactions when exposed to certain substances in their environments. Cats with *allergic dermatitis* (atopic dermatitis) develop skin disease characterized by signs of itching, including excessive licking and scratching at the skin when exposed to the material to which they have become allergic. You will often feel small bumps and scabs and sometimes see dandruff-like scales on the skin in affected areas in early cases. The skin may feel abnormally warm. Sometimes, however, signs go unnoticed until hair loss and broken hairs from excessive grooming are apparent. In neglected cases thickening of the skin accompanies hair loss. If they go untreated long enough, skin thickening and hair loss can become permanent. Areas where scratching, licking and chewing are severe may become infected.

Signs Of Allergic Dermatitis

Flea bites are probably the most common cause of allergic dermatitis. If you practice good flea control (see page 96), you may be able to prevent the dermatitis from developing or relieve a case which has already developed. Be careful, however, about putting flea sprays or dips on an irritated skin; they sometimes make the irritation worse. If you think you are controlling fleas, but your cat continues to have signs, there can be several possibilities, for example: 1) The bite of a single flea (which you may not see) can cause extreme irritation in an allergic animal. 2) Cats can be allergic to other things than or in addition to fleas — among them pollens and foods. 3) The condition may not be allergic dermatitis (see page 101 for an example).

Allergic Dermatitis Has Many Causes

A bath will help control the signs in many cats and can help control secondary bacterial infections. It removes allergens from the coat and seems to relieve some of the skin inflammation associated with allergic dermatitis. Use a gentle shampoo (e.g., baby shampoo, not bar soap or dishwashing detergent) to avoid additional damage to a sensitive skin. If your cat's skin and hair become too dry with bathing, Alpha-Keri® (one cap per quart of water) or some other

Bathing Is Part Of Home Treatment

122

non-toxic emollient oil can be used in the final rinse. If you find bathing makes your cat's skin worse or that it is too difficult to do, of course don't continue to use it as treatment.

Often once the itching has begun it continues even if you remove the original cause of the irritation. This may be due to scratching, which releases from the damaged cells substances that cause itching. When this cycle occurs a veterinarian must administer a corticosteroid (see page 212) to control the problem. In many allergic cats this treatment must be repeated intermittantly.

Skin testing and hyposensitization as used in people with certain allergies have been relatively unsuccessful in discovering the cause of allergies and treating them in animals. There are, however, veterinarians with special interest in skin disease who can make an effort to find out what your cat is allergic to in an attempt to relieve the problem. Ask your veterinarian for a referral if your cat has a skin problem which needs a specialist's care.

Contact Dermatitis

Contact dermatitis can occur in *any* cat whose skin comes into contact with an irritating substance such as certain soaps, detergents, paints, insect sprays or other chemicals. You will usually see reddening, red bumps and irritation of the skin which tends to be limited to the areas of contact with the substance and is more common in sparsely-haired skin areas. If left untreated, the affected areas may become moist and sticky.

Contact dermatitis is treated much like allergic dermatitis, but long term success is more likely since it is usually easier to find the offending substance and remove it permanently. The first thing to do is to remove the cause of irritation. If the contact dermatitis is due to a flea collar (see page 97), remove the flea collar. Bathe your cat and rinse the coat thoroughly. Then, if these steps are insufficient to relieve the signs, have a veterinarian examine your cat. Corticosteroids will probably be given and a soothing antibiotic-corticosteroid ointment dispensed, if necessary, for home use.

123

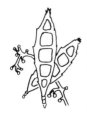

Ringworm (Dermatomycosis)

Ringworm is an infection of the skin caused by special types of fungus which may be transmitted via contact with spores to cats from other animals, people or the soil. Cats under one year old are more often affected than older animals. The "classic" sign of ringworm is a rapidly growing, circular area of hair loss, but it can appear in other ways — scaly patches, irregular hair loss, crust and oozing. A ringworm infection can be present with no evidence of skin disease.

Human Health Hazard

Certain kinds of ringworm can be transmitted from cats to humans. Adult humans are relatively resistant to ringworm, however, and are unlikely to become infected if normal clean habits, such as washing your hands and taking a bath regularly, are followed. Children should avoid handling animals infected with ringworm because they tend to be less sanitary and more likely to become infected.

Veterinarians can diagnose certain cases of ringworm with the use of an ultraviolet light alone (a certain type of ringworm fluoresces green). Microscopic examination of skin scrapings, and/or a fungal culture is often necessary in other cases. An inexperienced person may confuse ringworm with other skin conditions. If you are in doubt, see your veterinarian.

A cream or drops containing *tolnaftate* (Tinactin®) which is effective against ringworm can be purchased in the drugstore without a prescription. It will clear up a single infected area, but cannot be used to treat multiple spots or very large areas. It is best to combine topical treatment with the administration of *griseofulvin*. This drug is incorporated into new hair to prevent growth of the fungus. Your veterinarian will prescribe this drug (or perhaps something better as drugs change) when the diagnosis is made.

If your cat is diagnosed as having ringworm, clean your house thoroughly and wash or discard their bedding. The fungus forms spores (something like bread mold) and thorough cleaning helps remove them to prevent reinfection.

124

Feline Acne

Feline acne is a skin condition which occurs on the chin and edges of the lips in affected cats. In its mildest form you will see blackheads which may form in the skin because the cat does not wash the chin throughly and/or because of abnormal oil secretion of the skin glands in the area. When infection occurs, swelling of the chin may be seen and in severe cases actual pustules (pus containing bumps) or small abscesses form. Although mild cases of feline acne respond readily to treatment, you can expect recurrences when treatment is stopped since the underlying cause usually remains.

Home treatment consists of washing the chin of affected cats daily. Use a gentle soap (Phisoderm® or Phisodex® are good) and rinse thoroughly. Or gently scrub affected areas with rubbing alcohol (no need to rinse). Cases which don't respond to home treatment or chins which have become very infected will need to be treated with the help of a veterinarian who can prescribe antibiotics if necessary.

Rodent Ulcer (Eosinophilic Granuloma)

Rodent ulcer appears in several different ways in the skin of affected cats. The most common type of rodent ulcer is a reddish, raw looking area which occurs on the edge of one or both upper lips, most often in the area overlying the canine teeth. Although the surface looks eroded the skin in the area often feels thickened. Sometimes similar-looking lesions occur on the skin of the stomach, rear legs or feet, and lighter colored, more rough-surfaced affected areas are sometimes found inside the mouth. Although the cause of

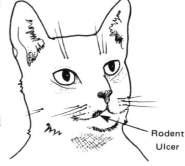

Rodent Ulcer

125

rodent ulcers is not known, it is thought to be related to prolonged irritation, such as that which may occur where the canine teeth rub against the lips or with prolonged and repeated licking of a skin area.

Rodent Ulcers Need Veterinary Attention

It is not possible to treat rodent ulcers at home without the aid of a veterinarian. Small areas which do not seem to irritate your cat may be left untreated, but most rodent ulcers enlarge slowly and eventually seem to cause discomfort or disability and need veterinary care. Some neglected lesions may become cancerous. Veterinarians treat rodent ulcers in several different ways. The treatment most often used is to inject corticosteroids directly into affected areas and/or prescribe them for oral administration at home. Measures which help prevent licking affected areas are employed, and in some cases surgical removal or x-ray therapy of affected areas is necessary.

Mastitis

Mastitis is an inflammation of one or more of the *mammary glands* (breasts) in female cats. While it may be due to abnormal drainage of milk from the gland, or to trauma, it is usually caused by infection. Affected glands look enlarged, may be discolored red, purplish or blue, and often feel hard and warm. They are often painful, making the female reluctant to let her kittens nurse. If you express some milk from the affected gland, it may be blood-streaked, pink, gray or brown. Often, however, the milk does not look unusual to the unaided eye. If left untreated, the gland may abscess or the female may develop more generalized signs of illness.

In order to prevent sick kittens, do not allow them to nurse from infected glands. Placing a piece of adhesive tape over the nipple of the gland will usually effectively prevent nursing. Affected glands should be milked out three to four times a day. Ask your veterinarian to show you how to do this properly. Warm packs applied to the gland seem to relieve discomfort and speed localization of infection. Infected glands must be treated with antibiotics. Your veterinarian will prescribe the appropriate ones.

126

Tumors (Cancer)

Tumors are often noticed as growths in, on or under a cat's skin. For more information turn to pages 165 and 186.

Umbilical Hernia

An *umbilical hernia* is a defect involving the body wall which is usually first noticed in young kittens as a lump under the abdominal skin. Its diagnosis and treatment are covered on page 246.

Virtually 98% of all the cats I see with signs of skin problems fall into one of the above categories. If you see signs you can't satisfy here, consult your veteriarian.

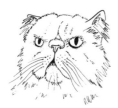

Head

EYES

General Information About Eyes

The eyes are very important and delicate organs. Mild and unobtrusive conditions can become severe rapidly, and many untreated conditions can cause irreversible damage. *Don't ignore even minor evidence of irritation.* Unless you are sure of the diagnosis and treatment, any minor eye problem which doesn't clear rapidly (within twenty-four hours) as well as any obvious change you see in the eye should be brought to the attention of an expert. DO NOT use anything in the eye not specifically labeled for *ophthalmic* use, and do not use a preparation in the eye just because you had it left over from an eye problem you or your cat had in the past. Ophthalmic drugs have very specific uses, and the use of a drug in a condition for which it was not specifically intended can cause serious injury or complication.

Epiphora (Tearing)

Epiphora is the abnormal overflow of tears from the eye. It has *many* causes because tearing is the eye's response to irritation. Among the causes are allergy, *conjunctivitis,* corneal injuries, and plugged tear ducts. In cats excessive tearing unaccompanied by other signs of illness is sometimes associated with mild upper respiratory infections (see page 135). In Persian cats, in particular, epiphora is mainly a cosmetic problem with no serious underlying physical cause. If you can eliminate other causes of tearing in these cats, staining of the fur can be controlled by frequent washing of the affected area and, if necessary, by clipping away stained hair.

Conjunctivitis

Conjunctivitis is an inflammation, sometimes caused by or accompanied by infection of the membrane which lines the lids and covers part of the eye (conjunctiva). It is

128

probably the most common eye problem of cats because it occurs in association with several of the common upper respiratory infections (see page 135) and also because the conjunctiva is exposed to so many irritants. The first sign of conjunctivitis may only be an increase in tearing with no other signs of irritation or illness. In many instances this type of conjunctival irritation will clear spontaneously in three to seven days. In other cases, the tearing changes or the first sign you notice is an excessive amount of sticky yellowish discharge which accumulates at the medial corners of the eye (see illustration page 22).

There are many degrees of inflammation. In mild cases the conjunctiva itself may look only slightly swollen or wrinkled. In more severe cases the conjunctiva is more pink than normal, sometimes very swollen and the vessels of the sclera (see page 23) are very prominent. Although mild conjunctivitis may clear without treatment, cases which are persistent, cause inflammation of the lids, and/or discomfort, or which are accompanied by other signs of illness must be treated by a veterinarian to avoid permanent damage to the eye.

In mild cases, the first step in treatment at home is to examine your cat thoroughly for other signs of illness and to examine the eyes thoroughly looking for a local cause of conjunctivitis to be removed if found. If there are no general signs of illness, if the eyes themselves look normal, and if the discharge is of the clear watery type, you may choose to postpone treatment for a few days. Cats with mild conjunctivitis which persists beyond seventy-two hours or which have a persistent sticky discharge, as well as those accompanied by other signs of illness, should be examined by a veterinarian who can determine whether antibiotics are necessary or who may find causes not obvious to you.

Conjunctivitis occurs frequently in kittens less than six weeks old. For more information see page 247.

For another cause of conjunctivitis, see Eyeworms, page 93.

Trauma To or Foreign Object In The Eye

Epiphora and conjunctivitis may be signs of a foreign body in the eye or eye injury due to trauma. So it's a good idea to examine your cat's eye thoroughly whenever there are such signs. If epiphora and/or conjunctivitis are *unilateral* (on one side) only, are accompanied by squinting, pawing at the eye or other signs of pain, a thorough examination for a foreign body or eye injury *must* be made.

The first thing to do when examining your cat's eye is to get in a good light. Slight, but extremely important, changes in the eye are easily overlooked in dim light. Place the thumb of one hand just below the edge of the lower lid of the affected eye and the thumb of the opposite hand just above the edge of the upper lid. This rolls the lids away from the eyeball allowing examination of the conjunctiva and most of the cornea. The surface of the cornea should look smooth and completely transparent. (If in doubt, compare it to the opposite, probably uninjured, eye.) Be sure to look along the edge of the third eyelid to see if there is anything protruding from behind it. It is a good idea to look under the third eyelid, but most cats with a painful eye will not allow you to lift this eyelid without some form of anesthesia. You can, however, moisten a cotton-tipped swab and move it *gently* along the inner surface of the lids and under the third eyelid. Occasionally a foreign body will cling to the swab and be removed, or the swab will sometimes bring a hidden foreign body into view. If you see a large object (e.g., foxtail), you can grasp it with your fingertips or a pair of tweezers and remove it. Small foreign bodies are most easily removed with a moistened cotton swab or a piece of tissue. Any foreign object not easily removed should be entrusted to a veterinarian, and *any* sign of irritation following foreign body removal which persists more than a few hours is reason

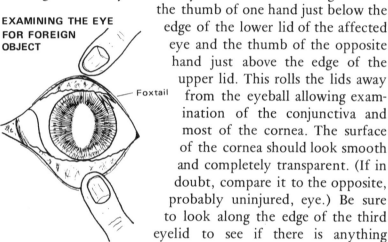

EXAMINING THE EYE FOR FOREIGN OBJECT

Foxtail

130

to have the eye examined by an expert.

I think in most cases of foreign body in the eye or trauma to the eye examination is best performed by a veterinarian. Since a cat can't tell you when there is eye irritation, it is often easy to overlook small but significant eye damage. Veterinarians use special eye stains to color the surface of the cornea. These stains show the presence of corneal damage not evident to the unassisted eye. Veterinarians also can give local or general anesthetics to relieve pain during examination allowing a more thorough search.

Prolapsed Third Eyelid

The third eyelid (nictitating membrane, see *Anatomy*, page 22) often moves from its normal position near the medial corners of the eyes to partially obscure the eye. When this occurs on one side only and intermittantly as if blinking, it is often a sign of local irritation to that eye, such as a foreign body or damage to the cornea. When it occurs in both eyes (often described by owners as a "film over the eye") and for prolonged periods of time (several hours to several days), it sometimes interferes with vision and can have many causes.

The most common cause of this second type of third eyelid elevation (third eyelid prolapse) in a cat which seems relatively healthy is a gastrointestinal upset. Signs which often accompany this kind of third eyelid prolapse are a change in appetite, a loose stool or vomiting. When the gastrointestinal disturbance is corrected, the third eyelids will return to their normal positions. Third eyelid elevation accompanied by more serious signs of illness (fever, weight loss, complete absence of appetite) should prompt you to have your cat examined by a veterinarian.

Third eyelid prolapse which occurs in an apparently healthy cat displaying no signs of illness (not even mild intestinal disturbance) is frequently without apparent cause. It usually disappears spontaneously. If you feel confident that your cat is healthy after performing a physical examination, you may then choose to wait and watch your cat for a few days in hopes that the problem will quickly correct itself. If prolapse is severe enough to interfere with vision, your veterinarian can supply you with a prescription for eye drops which will provide temporary symptomatic relief, if no evidence of general illness is found when they examine your cat.

EARS

External Ear Inflammation (Otitis Externa)

Otitis externa is a term used medically to describe an inflammation of the external ear (outside the eardrum). It has many causes, but the signs are usually the same. Head shaking and scratching at the ears are probably the most common. In some cases the cat will tilt their head slightly toward the side of the irritated ear, and touching it may cause signs of pain. Large amounts of waxy discharge are often present; in severe cases there may be actual pus. The inside of the pinna is sometimes abnormally pink and there may be swelling. (See *Anatomy* page 24 if you are not familiar with a normal cat ear.) The normal smell of a healthy cat ear becomes fetid as the inflammation gets worse.

The most common cause of otitis externa of cats is probably ear mites (see page 100). If you cannot be sure that ear inflammation in your cat is caused by mites or if you are not *sure* you can treat the problem at home, enlist the aid of a veterinarian. Ear inflammation not treated promptly and vigorously can result in ear changes which make conditions that could have been easily cured at first difficult or impossible to treat successfully, and the infection can progress to include the middle and inner ear. If you are unable to obtain the services of a veterinarian and don't think the ear problem is caused by ear mites or a foreign object in the ear (rare in cats) and choose to attempt home treatment, try using seventy percent isopropyl alcohol (rubbing alcohol). First clean out the affected ear (see page 201). Then twice a day, after a more minor ear cleaning, instill several drops of alcohol into the ear canal and massage the base of the ear to spread the medication all the way down the canal (see page

202). If you see improvement within three or four days continue treatment for two weeks. If there is no improvement or if the alcohol seems too irritating to your cat's ear, be sure to seek professional help.

Ear Swellings

Swellings on cats' ears are usually abscesses (see page 120). In a few cases they are *hematomas* (accumulations of blood under the skin) caused by trauma to the ear — such as excessive ear scratching and head shaking accompanying untreated otitis externa, or by fights. If there is no fever and the swelling is not draining, an abscess may be indistinguishable from a hematoma without examination of the contents by a veterinarian. Hematomas must be treated surgically by drainage and suturing to prevent deformity of the ear. If deformity is of no concern to you, you can allow a hematoma to heal on its own. Just be sure underlying problems such as ear infection are corrected.

NOSE

Important conditions involving the nose alone in cats are rare. A watery or sticky opaque white to yellow discharge from one or both nostrils is usually accompanied by sneezing and is a sign of more generalized illness, most often upper respiratory infection (see page 135).

MOUTH

Foreign Object In Mouth

Cats that have gotten foreign objects stuck in their mouths usually paw at their mouths and make unusual movements with their lips and tongues. They may make

133

gagging motions and drool, but do not always do so. Try not to get excited if you think your cat has something stuck in their mouth. Try to reassure and calm them, then perform a thorough mouth examination in good light (see page 27). Be sure to examine the areas of the mouth around the molars thoroughly; look under the tongue, at the soft and hard palates and far into the back of the mouth (pharynx). The most common objects you may find are sewing needles, pieces of string wrapped around the tongue or teeth, and small pieces of bone (e.g., splintered chicken bones). If you see the foreign body, grasp it with your fingertips or tweezers and remove it. If your cat is uncooperative or if you can't find anything, but the signs persist, you will have to have your cat examined by a veterinarian.

Dental Tartar

Dental tartar is hard white, yellow or brown material on your cat's teeth. For more information see *Anatomy* page 28 and *Preventive Medicine* page 56.

Gingivitis

Red or bleeding gums may be signs of gingivitis. See page 27 in *Anatomy* and page 57 in *Preventive Medicine* for more information. Gingivitis not responding to home treatment as discussed in these sections needs to be examined by a veterinarian. Some cats seem abnormally prone to gingivitis and some cases are difficult (sometimes impossible) to treat successfully even with expert veterinary help.

Respiratory System

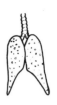

Feline Upper Respiratory Infections

Upper respiratory infections of cats are caused by numerous organisms. The most common are several different viruses and a bacterium-like organism (see table) which infect the tissues of the nasal cavity, eye and sometimes the mouth. All of these respiratory infections are contagious from cat to cat, some more extremely so than others, and they can range from very mild to very severe illnesses. They are probably the most frequently seen infectious diseases of cats. The important thing for you as a cat owner to know is not how to distinguish among the various upper respiratory infections (veterinarians often can't without refined laboratory tests), but how to prevent them, how to recognize that an infection is present, and how to determine when veterinary care is necessary.

Signs Of Upper Respiratory Infection

The most common signs of upper respiratory infection are sneezing, fever, watery to sticky, pus-like discharges from the nose and eyes, lack of appetite and listlessness. Sometimes drooling is seen, and in these instances raw areas *(ulcers)* can often be found on the tongue or hard palate. Some very mild infections are marked only by evidence of a mild eye irritation (conjunctivitis) accompanied by a small amount of watery eye discharge and no other signs. In severe cases the eyes can be swollen and crusted shut from discharges, the nasal passages clogged, the nose raw, and the cat most uncooperative with any efforts to aid them. In any one instance whether an upper respiratory infection is mild, moderate or severe is dependent upon many factors — among them, the age of the cat, their general health, their acquired resistance from previous exposure or vaccination and the strain of the infective organism.

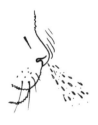

When To Seek Veterinary Help For URI

Upper respiratory infection in which the signs are mild — small amounts of watery eye and/or nose discharge and a few sneezes unaccompanied by fever — usually do not require veterinary care if the cat is eating normally (or near normally) and does not seem unduly depressed. Cases accompanied by any of the following signs should alert you

135

to have your cat examined by a veterinarian: persistent fever, lack of appetite, listlessness incongruous with other accompanying signs, dehydration, pus-like eye or nose discharges, or cough (a sign that the infection may have spread to include the lower air passages or that pneumonia may be present). Prompt and intensive treatment is necessary to avoid undesirable after effects of upper respiratory infections which are not mild.

Common Upper Respiratory Infections of Cats

Name of Disease	Disease Agent	Principal Signs	Comments
Feline Rhinotracheitis	Herpesvirus	Sneezing, coughing, eye and nose discharge, fever, drooling, lack of appetite, termination of pregnancy (abortion).	Usually severe infection of longer than one week's duration; can be fatal. Recovered cats may become carriers.
Feline Influenza	Picornavirus	Sneezing, eye discharge, lack of appetite, fever, ulcers on tongue, drooling.	More than fifteen different virus strains (like human colds). Symptoms vary from mild to severe. Recovered cats may become carriers.
Feline Pneumonitis	Clamydia sp.	Sneezing, watery eye discharge.	Usually mild infection. Responds to antibiotics. Strains of organism vary.
Feline Reovirus Infection	Reovirus	Watery eye discharge.	Usually very mild infection; often no treatment needed.

In most instances you will be responsible for the major portion of treatment of upper respiratory illnesses in your cat. Veterinarians are reluctant to hospitalize cases of upper respiratory infection unless absolutely necessary because many cats are "emotionally happier" at home, because these diseases are so contagious to other cats, and to avoid contamination of the hospital. The first step in home treatment of upper respiratory infection (even the most mild) is to keep your cat indoors. This protects them from the stress of temperature changes, prevents them from disappearing while sick, and also helps prevent transmission of the infection to other cats in the neighborhood. If possible, make an attempt to isolate your sick cat to prevent spread of the infection; change your outer clothes and wash your hands each time you medicate or handle the sick cat and provide separate food and water pans for the affected cat. These precautions are difficult in most household situations and in some instances impossible. If you own a cattery, such precautions are a must — ask your veterinarian for additional help. Further nursing care consists of keeping a daily temperature record (see page 192) and the administration of antibiotics (in most cases to control secondary bacterial infection which occurs after the cat is weakened by the original infection), decongestants, eye medications, and vitamins as directed by your veterinarian and hand feeding as necessary (see page 198). Since most sick cats do not groom themselves well, gentle removal of eye and nose crusts with a soft tissue or cotton ball moistened with warm water and daily brushing goes a long way in making a sick cat look and feel better. Cats which have extreme congestion of the nasal passages may benefit by the twice daily (no more) administration of ¼% acqueous phenylephrine nose drops (Neosynephrine® pediatric nose drops) into each nostril and by the use of a vaporizer for fifteen to thirty minutes about three times each day. (If you don't have access to a vaporizer you can run a hot shower until the bathroom is steamy and place your cat in the bathroom for fifteen to thirty minutes.) In upper respiratory infections treated at home it is often necessary to work closely with your veterinarian on an

137

outpatient basis. Injections of fluids to control dehydration and of antibiotics can be given as necessary, and periodic evaluation of your cat's progress can be made by an expert. Sometimes close cooperation between you and your veterinarian is not sufficient, and hospitalization is necessary.

After-Effects Of Upper Respiratory Infection Although prolonged treatment is necessary in severe cases of upper respiratory infection (more than two weeks in some), complete recovery usually occurs. Some cats (usually neglected cases or kittens) suffer permanent damage to the tissues lining the eye, sinuses or nasal passages. These cats may have a constant clear discharge from the nose and/or eye. Some with sinus disease have a recurrent or persistant cloudy discharge from the nose accompanied by sneezing and signs of nasal congestion. Cats left with such problems following upper respiratory infection are not always disabled but need examination and treatment by a veterinarian to determine whether the problem can be cured. Another after-effect of infection with upper respiratory disease is that many recovered cats remain carriers of the disease. Although apparently healthy, they can spread the infection to susceptible cats and when stressed (e.g., boarded away from home) may have milder recurrences of signs of infection.

Prevention The most severe problems with upper respiratory infections in cats are found where large numbers of cats are congregated together with inadequate sanitary precautions such as often occurs in boarding kennels, pet shops and catteries. Infections can be acquired in veterinary hospitals as well, but the problem occurs less often than in some other situations because veterinarians know and use all sanitary precautions available to avoid exposure of uninfected cats. The average pet owner can prevent feline upper respiratory infections by keeping their cat indoors, avoiding handling strange cats, and avoiding boarding their cat whenever possible. Catteries must follow special precautions to avoid contamination of premises or production of carrier cats. These include:

Sanitary Practices For Catteries 1) Only small groups of cats should be quartered together (less than ten) and each should have their own

138

separate pen placed so that it is impossible for one cat to sneeze on another. Cats should not be moved from pen to pen before the pen is thoroughly disinfected.

2) Quarters for cats should be well-ventilated but the temperature and humidity should be kept constant.

3) Isolation facilities should be provided. Sick cats should be removed from the cattery at the first sign of any illness and placed into the isolation area for the duration of their illness and for at least two weeks after recovery. All new cats to be introduced to the colony and all cats taken off the premises where they might be exposed to disease should be isolated for two weeks or more before introduction into the cattery.

4) Good sanitary practices should be followed to prevent the spread of disease-causing organisms which can travel via inanimate objects such as clothing and hands from cat to cat. These include thorough washing and disinfection of all food and water pans, thorough disinfection of all cage surfaces before transfer of a new cat into a previously occupied pen, changing outer clothing and thorough hand washing before feeding or handling healthy cats after treating sick cats or following exposure to cats not members of your cattery.

Vaccines are available against feline rhinotracheitis and feline pneumonitis. Feline pneumonitis vaccine has been available since the 1950's. Although once thought to be extremely effective in the prevention of pneumonitis, its efficacy is now questioned. The evidence indicates that the product available is not very (if at all) effective against field strains of the organism and the immunity produced is short-lived. Therefore its use is questionable. Feline rhinotracheitis vaccine is new to the market in 1974. Its benefits for cat owners will have to be determined following clinical use. Ask your veterinarian about its possible usefulness to you.

Vaccines Available

Chronic Allergic Bronchitis (Asthma)

Inflammation of the airways in the lung *(bronchitis)* can follow or accompany most respiratory diseases of cats. It is

139

also a response to inhaled infectious and irritant materials. In the common chronic bronchitis of cats, the inflammation of the airways seems to be an allergic reaction to inhaled allergens which is prolonged by repeated exposure to them. Affected cats usually seem healthy (no fever, eating well) but have intermittant bouts of deep, low-pitched, moist-sounding coughs. The affected cat usually sits with their shoulders hunched up, coughs several times and sometimes gags up foamy mucus-like material or swallows hard following each coughing bout. Often the problem is more severe certain times of the year than others. If left untreated, this condition sometimes progresses to *asthma*, in which the affected cat has attacks of extreme difficulty breathing (wheezing).

Although there is no permanent cure for feline chronic bronchitis of allergic origin and although signs of bronchitis are not emergency situations requiring immediate care, it is important to take your cat to see your veterinarian if you suspect this condition. Only your veterinarian can distinguish between chronic allergic bronchitis and other conditions which may cause similar signs (e.g., lungworms), and drugs designed to relieve the airway inflammation and thereby prevent asthma can only be prescribed by a veterinarian who has determined that it is safe to use them.

Laryngitis

Laryngitis is an inflammation of the larynx ("voice box," vocal cords) which causes a change of or loss of voice in cats. There can be many causes. Some cases are caused by infection (viral, bacterial); others are simply the result of excessive meowing (e.g., in Siamese cats). Laryngitis unaccompanied by fever or other signs of illness usually needs no treatment and clears within about five to seven days. Laryngitis which does not heal rapidly, is accompanied by signs of illness or which seems to cause excessive discomfort to your cat requires the help of a veterinarian.

140

Most respiratory diseases, if neglected, can progress to pneumonia or other serious conditions involving the respiratory system. Be sure to have your cat examined by a veterinarian in the presence of any of the following signs: persistant nose or eye discharge, difficult breathing, fever, or any signs you do not feel confident about.

For other causes of respiratory disease, see *Toxoplasmosis*, page 84, and *Lungworms*, page 92.

Musculoskeletal System
(Muscle and Bone)

General Information About Muscle and Bone Injuries

Musculoskeletal problems not related to injury are rare in cats. Diseases seen frequently in dogs such as hip dysplasia and patellar luxation which have a hereditary predisposition are almost never seen in cats; therefore you as a cat owner have little in the way of bony or muscular problems to consider when choosing a cat. Your problems with musculoskeletal disease will most likely arise following trauma to your animal.

Many musculoskeletal injuries can be difficult to diagnose, even by an experienced veterinarian. Proper diagnosis often requires the use of x-rays as well as a thorough physical examination. It may be impossible to distinguish among fractures, dislocations and sprains without the aid of x-rays. In general, however, it whould not be too difficult to distinguish the presence of a fracture or dislocation from the presence of a sprain, strain or bruise. Keep in mind that, although musculoskeletal injuries often cause marked signs, they themselves are not usually emergencies (see page 168). Review the musculoskeletal section in *Anatomy* page 11, then read this section thoroughly, and become familiar with your cat's normal posture and movement in order to prepare yourself to recognize any injury to your cat's muscles and/or bones.

When actual injury occurs, keep calm and proceed with an examination in a thorough and deliberate manner. First try to localize the site of the injury. To accomplish this, stand back and look at your cat as a whole. Try to determine the area (or areas) causing the change in posture or gait. If legs are involved, which are they? Which seem to hurt, look distorted or are being "protected" by the cat? Swelling is often fairly well confined to the injured area, but is sometimes extensive. The posture of an affected leg *may* be fairly normal above, but not below, the affected area. Once you have a general idea of the location of the problem examine each part of the limb, including each joint, gently

142

and carefully. All legs should be examined thoroughly, but you will probably want to go over the most obviously damaged one first. Review how to perform a leg examination in the anatomy section of this book if you feel unsure about it, and remember that comparing an injured leg to its (probably) uninjured mate can be very helpful.

Sprains, Strains, Bruises
Sprains, strains and bruises consist of damage to the soft tissues surrounding and supporting the bones. In these injuries swelling and signs of pain are often quite diffuse. They are not usually accompanied by fever. You may not be able to determine the exact site of injury, only the general area involved. If your cat has lameness due to a soft tissue injury, improvement will probably occur rapidly (two to seven days) with rest, and usually no other treatment is necessary. You may be tempted to give pain relievers, such as aspirin to your cat for such injuries: *avoid doing so.* Most human preparations are contraindicated in cats, and such drugs mask signs which are important in causing your cat to rest the injury and are important cues for you to use for gauging the degree of recovery.

Fractures
Complete fracture (break) of any of the major limb bones usually results in the *inability to bear weight* on the affected limb, and some *deformity* of the limb is seen. Deformity may consist simply of swelling, or include *angulation* (formation of an abnormal angle) usually at the fracture site, rotation or shortening of the affected limb, or other deviations from the normal position. The sound and feel of bone grating against bone *(crepitus)*, if present, is almost always indicative of a fracture. Unless sensory nerves have been damaged or the cat is in deep shock (see page 169), evidence of pain can be elicited by manipulating the fracture. Signs of pain, however, are unreliable since it can be present in other conditions as well, since many sensitive cats overreact to relatively mild pain, and "stoic" cats may be less likely to react strongly to painful stimuli.

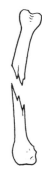

143

Fractures are classified as *simple* if there is no communicating wound between the outside of the skin and the broken bone. *Compound* fractures communicate to the outside. If your cat has a compound fracture with bone protruding from a wound, you should have no difficulty diagnosing the condition. Compound fractures easily become infected, and should be given immediate attention by a veterinarian if at all possible. If your cat is in fairly normal

FORELEG SPLINT

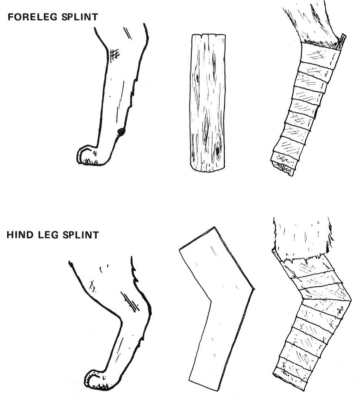

HIND LEG SPLINT

general condition, simple fractures are not necessarily veterinary emergencies. The best thing to do is to try to localize the fracture site, then call your veterinarian for further advice. Fractures of the foot bones are rarely emergencies and can usually be left unsplinted until x-ray pictures *(radiographs)* can be taken. Whether or not you splint other limb fractures depends on the site of the fracture and

144

the mobility of the bone ends. In most instances of limb fracture in cats, splinting causes more trouble for you and pain for the cat than it's worth. In an obviously mobile fracture, where you see the leg below the break dangling freely and twisting, heavy cardboard cut to the appropriate shape, roll cotton and elastic bandage can be used to prevent bone movement, interruption of blood supply and nerve damage until veterinary help can be obtained. Compound fractures should have a clean bandage applied over exposed bone ends if splinting is unnecessary.

A special case of fracture (or dislocation) is fracture of the spine. This situation requires professional veterinary care at the earliest possible time, and careful first aid. Spinal fractures usually result in partial or complete paralysis of the rear legs and sometimes the front legs as well, often with remarkably little evidence of pain. If your cat shows such signs following trauma, immediate and absolute (if possible) restriction of movement is necessary. Try to get your cat to lie quietly (but don't forcibly restrain them) and transport them in a box with high sides. Cats can be lifted and carried in your arms if you are careful to prevent back movement. *Spinal Fractures Are Emergencies*

The method a veterinarian chooses to repair a fractured bone depends on the type of fracture present, the fracture site, and the age of your cat. External devices alone, such as casts and splints, can be used in some cases. In many others surgery to place a metal pin, plate or other internal fixation device into the fractured bone is necessary. Good veterinarians will x-ray the fracture, evaluate all the possibilities for repair, and tell you what they think is necessary to achieve the best healing. If you cannot afford the best repair, they should offer alternative methods which may not be as ideal for healing but more within your means. (Keep in mind that the alternatives may mean slower healing or no repair at all.) *Fracture Repair*

Dislocations

Dislocations *(luxations)* are seen much less frequently than fractures in most veterinary practices. They occur whenever a bone is displaced from its normal contact with

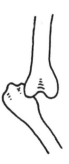

145

another bone at a joint. *The signs of dislocation are similar to those of fracture, but are usually milder.* Dislocations are not emergencies in the sense that they endanger a cat's life or limb. However, they should be examined by a veterinarian within twenty-four hours of occurrence because they are most easily corrected without surgery during this period. All suspected dislocations should be x-rayed to determine the true extent of bony damage. General anesthesia is given to relax the muscles and provide relief from pain while the bones are manipulated back into their proper positions. Some dislocations require surgery for permanent correction.

Nutritional Secondary Hyperparathyroidism (Paper Bone Disease)

Signs of this bone condition are seen most often in young growing kittens, but the basic changes in metabolism and bone which occur are induced in *any* cat fed a diet imbalanced in calcium and phosphorus. The cause of this nutritional bone disease is usually a diet which consists solely or primarily of meat (muscle or organs such as heart, kidney or liver). This results in an abnormally low calcium intake and abnormally high phosphorus intake (see page 64), and in turn stimulates the parathyroid glands to make metabolic adjustments in an attempt to return blood calcium and phosphorus to levels more nearly normal. Since insufficient dietary calcium is available to make the necessary adjustments, the skeleton is called upon to furnish it and demineralization of bone occurs.

Since the demand for calcium is particularly high in the first six to eight months of a cat's life, signs of paper bone disease are usually most marked in such animals. Bowing of the legs, abnormal spinal curvature and reluctance to move (a sign of pain) occur and have been misdiagnosed by some owners and veterinarians as "rickets." Spontaneous fractures may even occur, and if the condition is left untreated death may be the final result. Nutritional secondary hyperparathyroidism can be very deceptive. Because meat is high in protein and fat, kittens fed improper high meat or all meat diets can maintain a healthy appearance in terms of body

146

weight and normal hair coat while the bony changes are occurring.

Unless you have seen the disease before, you may have difficulty recognizing paper bone disease. Your veterinarian, however, should be able to diagnose it, and you will need veterinary expertise to treat it successfully. The best thing you can do as an owner is to prevent paper bone disease by feeding your cat (young or adult) a balanced diet (see page 58).

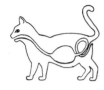

Digestive System
(Gastrointestinal Tract)

Vomiting

Vomiting is the *forcible* expulsion of stomach and/or intestinal contents through the mouth. It is important to try to distinguish between true vomiting and *regurgitation*, which is the *passive* act of returning the contents of the esophagus or pharynx through the mouth. This distinction will help your veterinarian make a diagnosis if home treatment is unsuccessful. Vomiting is a *sign* of various illnesses, not a disease in itself.

Vomiting occurs commonly in cats, and it is often accompanied by diarrhea. It seems to be caused most often by irritation of the stomach, which veterinarians call *acute* or *simple gastritis.* Gastritis is usually caused by the ingestion of an irritant substance — for example, decomposed food, grass, paper or bones. The cat often first vomits food or another irritant material, and later vomits frothy clear or yellow fluid. Cats with gastric irritation may seek grass to eat, but grass eating is often an "enjoyable pastime" for cats and not a sign of illness. They may or may not be interested in their normal food. If your cat vomits once or twice, has no fever or obvious abdominal pain and is no more than slightly depressed you can probably treat the vomiting at home.

Home Treatment For Vomiting

Do not feed your cat for the next twelve to twenty-four hours following vomition. At the end of twelve hours (if you can't stand to wait longer), you can offer a very small (about a tablespoonful) of soft, bland food such as a soft-boiled egg, baby food, cooked baby cereal or cottage cheese. If your cat keeps this small meal down for about four hours, another small meal can be offered, then another about four hours later. If no further vomiting occurs, the next day's meals can be normal-sized portions of bland food and the following day you can return your cat to a regular diet. Water or other liquids should be offered only in small amounts at one time. Large amounts of food or water distend the already irritated stomach and usually cause vomiting to recur. An easy way to have water available in small portions is to place ice cubes in the water bowl. This allows the cat to drink the liquid that

148

accumulates as the cubes melt.

Antacid liquids, (e.g., Maalox®, Mylanta®) or intestinal protectants such as Kaopectate® will help soothe the irritated stomach lining. Maalox® or Mylanta® can be given at a rate of one half teaspoonful per ten pounds body weight every eight hours until the signs have passed. If vomiting is present with diarrhea (gastroenteritis) Kaopectate®-like drugs are best (see page 151). Do not give any preparations containing aspirin.

Times To Seek Veterinary Help For Vomiting

If your cat vomits more than a few times, if the vomitus is ejected extremely forcefully (projectile vomiting), if there is blood in the vomitus or obvious abdominal pain, if your cat seems particularly depressed, weak or has a fever, or retches unproductively, DO NOT attempt to treat the condition at home. Even simple gastritis cannot always be treated successfully without the help of a veterinarian, and there are many other serious causes of vomiting, among them foreign objects in the digestive tract, panleukopenia (see page 78) and kidney failure (see page 187).

Some cats (particularly Siamese in my experience) vomit occasionally following meals. This type of vomiting is usually not serious in nature and may have several causes. Among the most common seem to be food gobbling, overeating or a particular sensitivity to certain kinds of food. If your cat is an after meal vomiter, trying one or more of the following things may help you:

1) If your cat eats with other animals, feed them alone. Not only offer an individual food bowl but feed them at a distance from the others. Competition encourages food gobbling.

2) Feed smaller meals more frequently.

3) Try a food which has to be chewed well before swallowing (e.g., dry kibbles instead of canned food).

4) See if you can associate the vomiting with the type of food fed. Some cats do better on dry food than when they eat the canned type. Sometimes you will find that it is only one brand or only one flavor which seems to cause the problem. If you do find a specific food which seems to be the cause, of course don't continue to feed it.

149

Hairballs   Hairballs can also cause vomiting of a non-serious nature, but sometimes they cause serious obstruction and must be removed surgically. When hairballs are vomited they usually are tubular, brown masses and are vomited by themselves or accompanied by a small amount of clear, foamy fluid. If you look closely at such masses or tease them apart you will find that they are composed primarily of hair. If you find vomited hairballs and your cat is acting normally you may assume that the current hairball problem is solved. This should alert you, however, to do something about hairball prevention to avoid future problems, as should stools which have a large amount of hair in them. A hairball problem can also cause lack of appetite or constipation.

Prevent hairballs by brushing your cat regularly and by the routine administration of commercial hairball prevention preparations available through your veterinarian or at pet stores. A home remedy for hairball prevention is mineral oil (or petroleum jelly). Other oils are not efficient hairball preventives because they are digested and absorbed by the cat. Add mineral oil at a rate of one teaspoonful per ten pounds body weight to the food once or twice a week for hairball prevention. (Petroleum jelly can be given directly. See page 152.)

Diarrhea

Diarrhea is the passage of abnormally soft and/or frequent stools. This *sign* is often associated with vomiting, but may be present alone. And it often causes cats to fail to use their litter pans. Diarrhea has many causes; the most common are dietary. All-meat diets or diets containing cow's milk (see page 59) often cause diarrhea. Rich or spicy tablescraps and decomposed food are other common offenders, but any food, including commercial diets, can cause diarrhea in certain cats. Intestinal parasites (e.g., worms) may cause diarrhea (see page 83). I see this rarely, however, except in kittens. Diarrhea can be caused by psychological stress, such as a trip to the veterinarians's office, or by new animals in the house, but this type usually subsides quickly and needs no treatment.

150

Home treatment for diarrhea consists of withholding food for twelve to twenty-four hours (so don't be too worried if your cat is not hungry at first), then offering a bland and easily digestible diet such as baby food, cooked chicken or cooked eggs, for three to five days. (Veterinarians can provide you with special foods for diarrhea.) An intestinal protectant and absorbent such as Kaopectate® (two teaspoonfuls per ten pounds body weight every six hours) should also be given. Look for the cause of the diarrhea and try to eliminate it.

Home Treatment For Diarrhea

Diarrhea which persists longer than twenty-four to thirty-six hours without improvement, bloody diarrhea, diarrhea accompanied by vomiting, fever, listlessness or lack of appetite or dehydration should not be allowed to continue without seeking help from a veterinarian. If you decide to take your cat to a veterinarian for treatment of diarrhea, try to bring a stool sample when you go. This can be very helpful in diagnosis and treatment of the problem. The color, composition and consistency of the stool are important, and an examination for parasites may have to be performed.

Times To Seek Veterinary Help For Diarrhea

Constipation

Constipation is the difficult or infrequent passage of feces. This *sign* occurs infrequently in healthy cats. Although it may be due to relatively simple things such as diet or excessive hair ingestion during self-grooming, when a well fed and well cared for young cat has recurrent bouts of constipation it is a cause for concern and warrants treatment by a veterinarian. Most normal adult cats have one or two bowel movements eacy day, but since each cat is an individual and diet has a great influence, a routine must be established for each. One day without passing a bowel movement is not a crisis.

If constipation is mild, a change in diet may relieve the problem. Canned foods containing large amounts of ground bone should be avoided; they can sometimes produce rock hard stools only a veterinarian can remove. Feeding dry cat food will help some cats who have trouble with mild constipation since most dry foods have more bulk (fiber)

Home Treatment May Help Mild Constipation

than canned foods do. Water added to the food may help and a meal of fresh liver is very laxative. Mucilose® and hydrolose are commercial preparations you can try: they are designed for humans to add bulk to one's diet and are sold in drugstores. If you find that you must add such preparations to your cat's diet frequently, discuss the problem with a veterinarian.

Mineral oil (one teaspoonful orally per ten pounds body weight), petroleum jelly (one teaspoonful given orally), or an infant glycerine suppository inserted into the rectum will sometimes relieve more severe constipation. They work by softening and lubricating the stool. Like all laxatives they should not be used on a continuous or frequently repeated basis without professional advice. Once or twice a day for two days should be sufficient to relieve constipation. Mineral oil interferes with the absorption of oil soluble vitamins and prolonged continuous use could cause vitamin deficiency as well as treatment-induced abnormal bowel function. Mineral oil should be administered in food. DO NOT attempt to force it orally; if inhaled, it can cause severe pneumonia.

Enemas Are Best Given By A Veterinarian

An enema may be necessary to relieve *impaction* of the colon (hardened stool lodged in the colon). This is best performed by a veterinarian who should give your cat a thorough physical examination before treatment. Fleet® pediatric enemas can be purchased in drugstores if the services of a veterinarian are unavailable. Insert the lubricated nozzle of the enema into the rectum and administer the Fleet® liquid at a rate of one ounce per ten pounds body weight.

Straining associated with bladder infection (see page 156) and with severe diarrhea and intestinal inflammation are often confused with constipation. Be sure you know what the problem is before attempting to treat it. (If necessary, insert a gloved and lubricated finger into the rectum to feel the stool.)

Flatulence (Gas, Farting)

Having a flatulent cat around is more of an inconvenience than a real medical problem. Excessive gas

152

formation unaccompanied by other problems can usually be controlled by changing the diet. With a little observation you can often find that flatulence occurs only when a specific flavor or brand of food is fed or only with certain types of tablescraps. Flatulence accompanied by diarrhea necessitates thorough physical examination and treatment directed towards resolving the diarrhea. When the stool becomes normal, flatulence often disappears.

Anal Sacculitis

Impaction of the anal sacs sometimes accompanied by infection is an infrequent problem in cats. The most common signs of anal sacculitis are scooting along the ground and excessive grooming around the anal area and tail base. Scooting in my experience is rarely a sign of worms. An unusual twitching of the skin over the back or surprise "attacks" at the tail base can sometimes be explained by overly full anal sacs. Signs of simple anal sac impaction can usually be relieved by expressing the contents of the sacs. You can do this yourself. Use one hand to hold up the cat's tail. Hold a disposable cloth or tissue in the other hand. Place your thumb externally over one anal sac and your fingers over the other. Press in and apply firm pressure over the sacs. This causes the contents to be expressed out through the anus into the tissue so they can be discarded.

EXPRESSING THE ANAL SACS

Anal Sac Abscesses

If impacted anal sacs are not emptied, one or both may become infected. Infected sacs may be painful, and you may be able to express blood-tinged material or pus from the sac. If you don't notice the problem at this stage, you may later see an abscess or swelling externally at one side or the other of the anus. Infected anal sacs are best treated by a veterinarian. If they have not yet abscessed, it may be possible to treat them with

153

antibiotics alone. If they are abscessed, surgical drainage is usually necessary.

Obesity

Obesity (fatness) is almost always an owner-induced disease in pets caused by overfeeding. Excess fat puts excessive stresses on your cat's joints, heart and lungs and often results in an inactive cat. An obese cat, as you may have discovered, is more difficult to examine thoroughly than a normally-fleshed. one, since excess fat interferes with listening to or feeling the heartbeat, and with feeling the pulse and abdominal organs. An obese cat is a poorer surgical risk. If your cat is overweight, have them examined by a veterinarian if you want to be sure that their general health is good and that their condition is not caused by a medical problem, then put them on a diet.

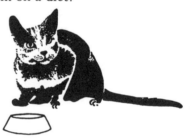

Desired Weight	Daily Maintenance Calorie Requirement (Tomcats require ten calories more per pound body weight)
4 lbs.	160
5 lbs.	200
6 lbs.	240
7 lbs.	280
8 lbs.	320
9 lbs.	360
10 lbs.	400
11 lbs.	440
12 lbs.	480
13 lbs.	520
14 lbs.	560
15 lbs.	600

Choose the weight you want your cat to reduce to. Then feed *fifty* to *sixty percent* of the daily Calorie requirement until the desired weight is reached. This could take several weeks. You can use the following as a guide to how much commercial food will provide the proper amount of Calories:

Type of Food	Approximate Calories per ¼ pound (4 ounces) Food
Dry	400
Semi-moist	400
Canned	125

If you make your cat's food, you will have to determine the Calorie content yourself. You can feed the calculated amount of food in as many meals as you desire each day, but, remember, *more food is not allowed* and be sure to include Calorie values for any "tidbits" fed.

Weigh your cat weekly. If you are following the rules set out above and your cat is not losing weight, consult your veterinarian for further help. Once your cat has reached the desired weight you can relax the rules a little to increase your cat's Calorie intake to the maintenance level for that weight.

An example: Your cat weighs twelve pounds, but should weigh nine. The daily maintenance Calorie requirement for a nine pound cat is about 360 Calories x 60% = 216 Calories to be fed while reducing. This is about 2.2 ounces dry or semi-moist food, or about 7 ounces of canned diet. After the desired weight is achieved, feeding could be increased to about 3.6 ounces of dry or semi-moist food or 11.5 ounces of canned food.

(When using a diet of commercial foods for weight reduction, consider providing your cat with a vitamin-mineral supplement. See *Nutrition* page 69 for more information.)

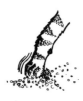

Genitourinary System

General Information

If your cat has any of the following signs, genitourinary (reproductive or urinary) system disease may be present and thorough examination by a veterinarian is indicated:

Drinking increased amounts of water

Urinating very frequently

Urinating abnormally large or small amounts

Difficulty or inability to urinate

Bloody urine

Blood and/or pus-like material dripping in quantity from the penis or vulva

Abdominal pain or walking with an abnormally arched back

Feline Cystitis-Urolithiasis Complex

Signs Of Bladder Inflammation Or Urinary Blockage

The cystitis-urolithiasis complex is the most common urinary tract problem seen in cats. Signs of *cystitis* (bladder inflammation and/or infection) most often include bloody urine and frequent urination of small amounts, sometimes accompanied by excessive licking at the genitals. Many times an affected cat will urinate in abnormal places inside the house such as the bathtub or shower or begin urine spraying (see page 161). Cases affected with severe *urolithiasis* (mineral crystals, tiny "stones" in the urine) may become completely blocked with sandy material and be unable to urinate (an emergency situation). Cases of complete urinary obstruction which go unnoticed or untreated progress to depression and weakness, dehydration, vomiting and eventually total collapse, coma and death. Even if treated, cases of urinary obstruction in the later stages may not recover. Body changes due to uremia (excessive retention of toxic wastes normally excreted by the kidneys) and kidney damage are sometimes irreversible.

Most veterinarians agree that several factors interact to produce a cystitis and/or urolithiasis problem in a cat.

156

Viruses, diet, water intake, patterns of urination, stress, bacteria and heredity all have been implicated, but veterinarians disagree as to which factors are most important in producing and controlling the illness. Viruses which produced urinary obstruction in exposed cats have been isolated, and they appear to be the likely culprits necessary to initiate the disease. But how these agents are transmitted and what other factors interact with them to produce the disease as it is usually seen have not yet been fully elucidated. Bacteria are isolated occasionally from cases of bladder inflammation and urinary obstruction in cats. If not eliminated they can be responsible for retrograde infection of the kidneys and permanent damage to the urinary system, but more often than initiating the problem, they are secondary invaders which become established after the urinary system has already been damaged. Until the complex etiology of this problem is worked out, there will be no reliable methods which an owner can follow to prevent the occurrence of cystitis and accompanying urolithiasis in their cat.

If you think your cat has signs of cystitis, try to get a look at the urine and examine the cat thoroughly. Straining associated with cystitis can easily be confused with straining accompanying constipation or severe diarrhea and vice versa so you need to do something to try to make sure what the exact problem is. If your cat has been urinating in abnormal places such as a sink or the bathtub, it may be easy to see whether the urine looks blood-tinged. Otherwise a small urine sample can be obtained at home by placing an open plastic bag over the litter in the litter pan. Blood-tinged urine almost always confirms the presence of severe bladder irritation and indicates that your cat should be examined by a veterinarian who can perform a complete urinalysis, determine whether bacteria are present and prescribe medication as necessary. Cystitis may be present when urine looks normal to you. In these instances only a urinalysis will confirm the condition's presence.

If your cat shows signs of cystitis but you cannot be sure urine is being passed, immediate physical examination

157

by you or your veterinarian is necessary to determine whether or not urinary obstruction is present. Urinary obstruction is *rare* in females; their broad urethras are not easily plugged by sandy material. It almost always occurs in males (both castrated and uncastrated) whose narrow urethras become blocked quite easily. Knowing this may help you with diagnosis. Feel for the bladder (see page 34). In obstructed cats, it can be felt as a lemon-sized or larger hard object and the cat (unless very depressed) will usually react as if in pain. (Unobstructed cats with cystitis who have urine in their bladders often urinate when you feel for their bladder.) Look at the penis. It is often extended beyond the prepuce; if it isn't visible, expose it (see page 32). In obstructed males its tip is often bloody and/or bruised looking, and sometimes a bit of white, sandy material can be protruding from the urethra. If you conclude that your cat is obstructed or cannot be sure that he isn't veterinary help is imperative. Only in instances of veterinary unavailability should you waste time attempting to relieve the obstruction yourself. If a veterinarian is absolutely not available, you can try the following:

A Veterinarian's Help Is Important In Cases Of Obstruction

1) Use firm but gentle manipulation of the penis to try to squeeze the obstructing material from the urethra. Try rolling the penis between your fingers working from nearest the body to the tip, and try milking the penis from its base to its tip. If your motions are being effective, gritty feeling, white or blood-tinged material will be expressed like toothpaste from the end of the penis. If you relieve the obstruction completely, urine will usually begin to flow freely from the penis.

"Sand"

2) If you remove some sandy material but urine doesn't flow, then try squeezing the bladder *gently* (you can rupture it if you aren't careful). This will sometimes result in a free flowing stream of urine.

An obstruction relieved at home still requires veterinary care if at all possible. Acutely obstructed cats tend to become plugged again and most cats docile enough to allow you to manipulate their penis and distended bladder need the specilaized supportive care only a veterinarian can give.

Veterinarians have many techniques for relieving obstruction. Unless the cat is extremely depressed, most administer general anesthesia, and once the obstruction is relieved, often a *catheter* (tube) is sutured in place and left for a few days to assure that the cat remains unblocked. Fluid therapy is administered to correct dehydration, stimulate a free urine flow and to remove toxic wastes from the body. Blood tests (to measure uremia) are often necessary. As in cats with uncomplicated cystitis, urinalysis will be performed and appropriate medications administered and dispensed for home use.

The most common drugs used in treatment of bladder inflammation and blockage are urinary acidifiers, antispasmodics and antibiotics. Antibiotics are useful only if bacteria are present in the urine and against bacteria which invade the cat's body secondary to the stress of the bladder problem. Antispasmodic drugs are used to relax the smooth muscle of the bladder and urethra in an attempt to prevent re-obstruction and to provide relief from discomfort. Urinary acidifiers are drugs which, as their name suggests, help promote the production or urine with an acid pH instead of an alkaline one. (Crystals responsible for urinary obstruction form in larger amounts in alkaline urine other things being equal.) Although antispasmodics and antibiotics are usually discontinued as signs of the acute stages have passed, urinary acidifiers often remain to be used on a long term basis in an effort to prevent recurrence of the problem. One of the best and most often used is *d-l*-methionine which your veterinarian will supply or which you can purchase in pet stores in products designed to help control the odor of cat urine. Measures other than urinary acidifiers designed to help prevent recurrent problems of urinary obstruction all involve the management of your cat at home.

Home Treatments To Prevent Urinary Obstruction

1) Be sure to encourage adequate water intake by providing fresh water readily available at all times. Water

intake can be increased fifty to one hundred percent by adding ordinary table salt to the cat's food at no more than one percent of the diet (a pinch per can of cat food is fine). Also add water to dry food if it comprises a large part of your cat's diet. An adequate water intake encourages good urine flow, and as more urine is produced any crystalline material present becomes less concentrated.

2) Feed a diet low in ash; the excessive mineral content of high ash diets may contribute to crystal formation. Canned food containing more than 3.5 percent ash (wet weight, check label) should not be fed. Also avoid any foods containing large quantities of ground bones (e.g., many fish products) and restrict or prohibit milk intake. (If milk is given, offer only small amounts and dilute it fifty percent with water.) Well-balanced commercial canned cat food which is low in ash is available through veterinarians and is an ideal product to feed.

3) Avoid dry cat foods. Although the role of dry cat foods in producing obstructions is very unclear, in controlled studies, feeding dry foods was shown to increase crystal formation as compared to a commercial low ash diet. It was theorized that this was due to poor water intake with dry foods and/or the high ash content *as compared to the control diet.* Dry foods are comparable or contain *less* ash (on a dry weight basis) than most canned foods available in supermarkets. So if you are going to continue to feed supermarket foods, adding water to dry foods may benefit your cat as much as feeding only canned foods with less than 3.5 percent ash. However, if your cat has severe problems with crystal formation, the best advice is to avoid dry foods and feed prescription low ash diets available from your veterinarian or made up at home.

4) Provide a litter pan that is clean and dry at all times. Many cats are so fastidious that they will hold their urine rather than use a litter box they consider too soiled. Other cats will hold their urine for long periods of time to avoid going outside to urinate in inclement weather. This causes urinary stagnation which is thought to contribute to crystal precipitation.

160

Even with the best home treatment, cats with cystitis-urolithiasis problems often have recurrent bouts of bladder inflammation or obstruction. It is impossible for your veterinarian to predict whether your cat's condition will be a one time problem or a recurrent nuisance. Veterinarians can only confirm the condition and make sure no other complicating problems are present. Simple feline cystitis (unaccompanied by bladder infection, bladder stones, or tumors) in female cats is more of an inconvenience for you and your cat than a life-threatening medical problem since recurrences usually cause only signs of bladder irritation. Recurrent urinary obstruction in male cats, however, is a serious and life-threatening situation. A good alternative to constant worry over the threat of obstruction is a surgical procedure called a *perineal urethrostomy.* In this surgery the small urethra of the male is enlarged so it no longer easily becomes blocked with sandy material. Although this surgery cannot cure the underlying problem, in the hands of a good veterinary surgeon its success rate is high and it solves the problem of worry and the repeated expense of treatment for urinary obstruction.

Surgery Can Help A Cat With Repeated Urinary Obstruction

Urine Spraying

Urine spraying is the act of squirting or spraying urine on vertical surfaces in response to territorial stimuli. This is a normal, but usually undesirable, behavior for unneutered adult, male cats (see page 226). It can usually be prevented or arrested by castration. Female cats and castrated males who have never sprayed before sometimes start spraying (or normally urinating abnormal places) at an advanced age. Usually this occurs as the result of some environmental change, such as the presence of a new cat in the house or some other environmental upset. It may, however, be associated with urinary tract disease, such as cystitis.

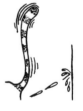

The best course of action to follow when a cat suddenly starts abnormal urination behavior, such as spraying, is to have the cat examined by a veterinarian who can perform a complete urinalysis. If physical examinations and urinalysis reveal no abnormalities, then you can work together in an attempt to find and solve the behavioral problem.

False Pregnancy
For signs of false pregnancy see page 231.

Uterine Infection
Pyometra

Pyometra is a type of uterine infection which occurs most commonly in older unspayed (or partially spayed, see page 224) females. It occurs most often in females who have never had a litter and is probably due to a hormonal imbalance. In cases of pyometra where the cervix is open there is usually a sticky reddish to yellow, pus-like, abnormal smelling discharge from the vulva. *Other cases have no discharge.* A female with pyometra is often listless, lacks appetite and may show increased water intake and increased urination. She may vomit and *sometimes* has fever. If not treated, this condition can cause death. *Ovariohysterectomy* (spaying) is the treatment of choice for pyometra. Cats treated without surgery often do not recover, and if they do recover, recurrences are frequent. Females with pyometra are much poorer surgical risks than healthy young cats, so consider having an ovariohysterectomy (see page 221) performed when your cat is young, and rush your cat to a veterinarian if you think pyometra may be present.

Acute Metritis

A retained placenta or fetus, or a lack of cleanliness during delivery can result later in an infection of the uterus, *acute metritis*. It may also follow or accompany spontaneous abortion. A female with acute metritis is usually depressed, febrile, lacks appetite and may seem uninterested in her kittens. She may seem excessively thirsty, vomit, and/or have diarrhea. The discharge from the vulva is often odorous, reddish and watery, or later, dark brown and pus-like. This condition calls for immediate treatment by a veterinarian. Kittens may have to be raised by hand (see page 243) since females with acute metritis often do not have enough milk, or the milk produced may be toxic.

162

Heart and Blood
(The *Cardiovascular* System)

Anemia

Anemia is a common sign of illness in cats. Anemia occurs whenever *a fewer than normal number of red blood cells* is circulating in a cat's blood stream. It has many causes. A borderline degree of anemia may only be recognized by your veterinarian with the help of a blood cell count or other laboratory tests. More pronounced anemia causes other signs which you may be able to recognize at home. Pale colored mucous membranes (look at your cat's gums, tongue, roof of *Signs of* the mouth and conjunctiva), decreased activity and decreased *Anemia* appetite usually accompany anemia in cats. An unusual accompanying sign seen in many anemic cats is an appetite for abnormal foodstuffs; many are seen to lick sidewalks or earthenware pots; others consume kitty litter. When anemia becomes very pronounced, pale mucous membranes become white, an abnormal "shh" sound may be heard in the heart beat (a *heart murmur*), complete loss of appetite usually occurs and any physical activity may lead to complete collapse and rapid, strained breathing. Also loss of bladder and fecal control is often seen. Anemia left untreated in these stages almost invariably becomes fatal within a few days or hours. If you recognize signs of anemia in your cat, seek the help of a good veterinarian. Discovery of the presence of anemia is only the first step; good treatment directed at the cause of the low red blood count requires thorough investigation. Rational therapy can only be applied when the specific disease producing the anemia is identified. Repeated *Kinds* blood counts and other more refined diagnostic tests, *Of Anemia* including measures of organ function (e.g., liver and kidney function tests) and bone marrow biopsy (removal of a sample of bone marrow for examination) are frequently necessary when treating an anemic cat. Patience and cooperation on your part are important assets if this serious problem arises.

The causes of anemia fall into three categories: anemia due to blood loss, anemia due to increased destruction of red blood cells, and anemia due to decreased production of new

163

red blood cells. Blood loss most often follows trauma, such as that which occurs when a cat is hit by a car (see page 171) or falls from a height. In cases of blood loss due to trauma, other evidence of injury is often present. Increased destruction of red blood cells usually accompanies *Hemobartonella felis* infection, *Feline Infectious Anemia.* This microscopic rickettsial organism attaches to the surface of the red blood cells causing them to be identified as abnormal and removed from the circulatory system. The organism responsible for this disease may be transmitted from cat to cat during fights, or through the uterus before birth. Blood-sucking external parasites such as fleas, lice and ticks may also be responsible for its spread. Carrier cats may be infected without showing signs of disease, and the exact combination of factors necessary for *Hemobartonella* to produce significant anemia is not yet fully understood. There are no preventive measures available for control of infectious anemia. The task of diagnosis and treatment requires the help of a veterinarian. The infectious anemia organism is often present accompanying other causes of anemia. In many of these instances treatment fails since antibiotic therapy directed at *Hemobartonella* may not help correct other more significant causes.

Feline Infectious Anemia

The failure to produce enough red blood cells is the more common cause of anemia in cats. This type of anemia is called *bone marrow depression,* but identifying an anemia as such is only a small part of the total picture. Cats have a very sensitive bone marrow and almost any chronic disease can cause bone marrow depression and resulting anemia. Anemia due to bone marrow depression accompanies disease processes as diverse as bacterial infection following fighting wounds, kidney failure, panleukopenia (see page 78), nutritional deficiencies, leukemia and lymphosarcoma (see below). Some causes are simple to diagnose and easy to treat; others are difficult to diagnose and sometimes impossible to treat successfully. In many instances the true problem emerges only after time passes and initial treatments do not succeed.

Treatment of anemia varies, of course, depending on its

164

cause. Drugs commonly employed are antibiotics and vitamin-mineral supplements. Bone marrow stimulants and blood transfusions are sometimes necessary as well. Home nursing care is very important. In addition to administering drugs as directed, you will need to provide a balanced diet and a warm, unstressful environment.

Leukemia-Lymphosarcoma Complex

The leukemia-lymphosarcoma complex consists of a controversial group of fatal diseases of the blood-forming organs, blood cells and lymphoid tissues (e.g., lymph nodes). These neoplasms (cancers) occur much more frequently in cats than in other animals and are the most common types of cancerous conditions seen in cats. Broadly defined, the *leukemias* are disorders of the blood-forming cells *(myeloproliferative diseases)* which are reflected by changes seen primarily in the blood and which are sometimes diagnosed only with great difficulty. Cats affected with such blood-forming disorders often show signs such as progressive weight loss, poor appetite, fever and pale mucous membranes (anemia). Since such signs often accompany other serious, but treatable diseases (e.g., feline infectious anemia, page 164), and since laboratory tests are imperative for diagnosis, it is obvious that a veterinarian's help is necessary if you suspect such a problem in your cat.

Lymphosarcoma (malignant lymphoma) is the most common tumor (abnormal growth of tissue) in cats. The solid growths (cancers) it produces have been found in almost every organ and tissue of cats, and the signs of its presence depend on the site of tumor formation. The most common site of cancerous growth is the abdomen; here kidney involvement may produce signs of kidney failure (see page 187); persistent diarrhea, constipation, and/or vomiting may occur with intestinal or lymph node involvement. Malignant lymphoma also is seen frequently in the chest, resulting in fluid formation, compression of the windpipe, and signs of respiratory diseases such as difficult breathing and coughing. Generalized lymph node enlargement occurs in other cases. Liver and spleen tumors can occur, and when tumor

165

formation occurs in unusual sites (e.g., brain, spinal chord, skin, eyes) the accompanying signs may be bizarre. Blood abnormalities (leukemia) may or may not accompany the solid tumor formation of lymphosarcoma.

Virus Is Found In Feline Leukemia And Lymphosarcoma

A feline leukemia virus, an *oncornavirus* (tumor producing, ribonucleic acid virus) has been isolated from cats with lymphsarcoma and blood-forming disorders. Many veterinarians now accept this virus as the cause of the feline leukemia-lymphosarcoma complex, and it is the source of much controversy among veterinarians and cancer researchers. One of the main disagreements concerns whether and how the cancer virus is transmitted from cat to cat. For example: one group feels that the virus may be transmitted genetically from parent to offspring. Another group feels that the virus can be transmitted directly from cat to unrelated cat and has shown that the virus can be shed in saliva and urine. Neither group can state what factors other than the presence of the feline leukemia virus are necessary for the development of disease and both agree that there is no evidence to indicate transmission of the virus from cats to humans or other animals. As a cat owner this disagreement is of little importance to you unless your cat develops leukemia or lymphosarcoma, or unless your cat associates with a cat which develops one of these serious diseases. In such instances it is best to discuss the situation thoroughly with your own veterinarian and decide what steps to take based on your individual circumstances and the most current information available.

Since the leukemia-lymphosarcoma complex can mimic so many other diseases and vice versa, any persistent signs of illness in your cat should prompt you to consult your veterinarian. Diagnostic techniques including complete blood counts, x-ray pictures, biopsy (removal of a piece of organ for examination), examination of chest and/or abdominal fluids and bone marrow examination are often necessary to confirm leukemia-lymphosarcoma or to exclude them from the diagnosis. A laboratory test which can identify the presence of feline leukemia virus in the white blood cells is now available. It can be a valuable aid to your veterinarian

Cancer Diagnosis May Need Extensive Testing

166

when they are attempting to determine whether or not leukemia or lymphosarcoma is present. A positive test, however, does *not* in itself indicate that an infected cat is ill with leukemia and/or lymphosarcoma. Frequently, repeated examinations and many days of observation are necessary before the final diagnosis can be made.

Leukemia and lymphosarcoma in cats are invariably fatal diseases. Treatment which your veterinarian can provide is directed at prolonging an affected cat's comfortable life. There are no specific home treatments, but, after knowing all the facts, if you decide to treat an affected cat your veterinarian can instruct you in supportive care and provide you with corticosteroids, antibiotics, vitamin-mineral supplements and anticancer drugs as necessary. At some point, euthanasia is often the most humane step to take (see page 189). New cats may be introduced into a household formerly occupied by a cat affected with leukemia or lymphosarcoma one month following house cleaning and disposal of litter pans, feed dishes and bedding used by the sick cat.

Heart Failure

Heart disease and accompanying heart failure is not a common problem in cats. When heart failure does occur it is seen most often in older cats. For more information see *Geriatric Medicine* page 188.

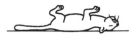

Emergency Medicine — First Aid

General Information About Emergencies

An *emergency* is any situation which requires immediate action in order to prevent irreversible damage to or the death of your cat. Each of the following signs indicates an emergency situation:

Uncontrollable bleeding
Extreme difficulty breathing
Continuous or recurrent convulsions
Unconsciousness
Shock
Sudden paralysis
Inability to urinate
Repeated or continuous vomiting and/or diarrhea

Conditions such as injury to the eyeball or snakebite are usually emergencies; others, such as possible leg injuries, are not so clear cut. Therefore, in many cases you will have to use your intuition to make a good judgement about the best action to take.

It is to both your and your veterinarian's benefit that you can accurately recognize an emergency. No veterinarian I know enjoys being taken away from dinner, pulled from the bathtub or awakened in the middle of the night by an hysterical pet owner who obviously does not have an emergency. Most veterinarians value their leisure time more than any emergency fee they may collect. And rational pet owners are often unhappy to find out upon reaching the veterinary hospital that the "emergency" could have safely waited until morning and that the emergency fee could have been saved. Usually getting emotionally upset leads to restricted judgement. Try to remain calm and use this section as a reference for making that emergency decision.

Most emergencies I see are the result of trauma (hit by a car, bitten by a dog) or poisoning. Most could have been easily prevented if the owner had confined their pet when unable to supervise them. Medical emergencies due to failure of a vital organ could often have been prevented by consulting a veterinarian soon after the earlier signs appeared. Look ahead. If a weekend or holiday is coming up, it may be a good idea to take your cat in for an examination even if the signs seem minor.

Shock

The term *shock* is one I hear frequently abused. It is extremely important to know whether or not shock is truly present, because its presence or absence often determines whether or not a condition is an emergency. Shock can be simply defined as *the failure of the cardiovascular system to provide the body tissues with oxygen.* There are several causes of shock; the most common in veterinary medicine is blood loss. The following are signs which may indicate the presence of shock:

1. Depression (quietness and inactivity) and lack of normal response to external environmental stimuli.

2. Rapid heart and respiratory rate.

3. Poor capillary refilling time. To test for capillary refilling time, press firmly against the gums, causing them to blanch (whiten) beneath your finger. Lift your finger away and see how long it takes for the color to return to the blanched area. The normal refilling time is no more than one or two seconds. Poor capillary filling is an early and constant sign in shock. It precedes the pale, cool mucous membranes present in more advanced shock.

4. Rapid pulse which becomes weak and may become absent as shock progresses.

5. Lowered body temperature. The extremities (legs and paws) and skin become cool to the touch and rectal temperature often drops below 100 degrees F.

If your cat shows signs of shock following injury or prolonged illness, contact a veterinarian immediately. But first wrap your cat in a towel or blanket (if possible) to preserve body heat.

Signs Of Shock Progressively More Serious

169

External Bleeding and How To Stop It (Hemostasis)

Most cuts through the skin will stop bleeding within five or six minutes of their occurrence. Those which do not or which are bleeding profusely need some kind of immediate care, especially if it's going to be a while before you can enlist professional veterinary aid.

How To Use A Pressure Bandage   A *pressure bandage* is the best way to stop bleeding. If a gauze pad is available, place this directly over the wound; then apply the bandage over it. Any clean strip of material can be used for a bandage. Gauze roller bandage, a strip of clean sheet or an elastic bandage are best since persistent

APPLYING A PRESSURE BANDAGE TO THE TAIL

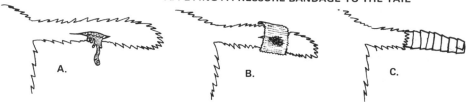

A.   B.   C.

bleeding causes seepage which you can see through such bandages. If the wound is on the trunk or you only plan to bandage a limb temporarily, apply several wraps of bandage firmly and directly over the wound. If the bandage is to be left on a limb for several hours or more, it should be applied over the wound and down the leg to cover the foot as well. This will prevent swelling and *ischemia* (lack of blood and oxygen) of the part of the limb below the bandage. This rule applies to bandaging the tail too. If you cannot apply a pressure bandage, firm *direct pressure* (with your bare hand, if necessary) over the wound for several minutes will often stop bleeding.

If a pressure bandage will successfully stop the bleeding and no other problems are apparent, you can usually wait until the next day to have the wound examined and treated by a veterinarian. Most wounds severe enough to require a pressure bandage will need *suturing* (sewing closed) for proper and most rapid healing. (Any wound which gapes open is likely to benefit from suturing.) Use your judgement as to whether the need for stitches is immediate.

A *tourniquet* is a second and *much less desirable*

170

method of achieving hemostasis. Tourniquets are useful only for bleeding involving a limb or the tail. They should be loosened *at least* every fifteen minutes to allow reoxygenation of tissues. Use any strong cord, rope or bandage strip to form a tourniquet. Form a loop and apply it on the extremity between the body and the wound. (It is easiest to apply it at a joint to prevent slippage.) Watch the change in blood flow to determine how tightly to tie the tourniquet. Proper application will usually cause an immediate and definite slowing of blood seepage. When you achieve sufficient slowing, stop tightening the tourniquet. (Don't expect a completely blood free area.) Then consider replacing the tourniquet with a pressure bandage if at all possible.

How To Apply A Tourniquet

Hit By A Car

The first thing to do if you find your cat hit by a car is try to remain calm. This isn't easy since your animal is so important to you, but hysterics will not help you or your cat. Try to assess the damage that has been done. You must gather information to help your veterinarian decide the seriousness of the injuries before you get to the hospital. So concentrate on this plan of action while adminstering first aid.

Many seriously injured animals try to run from the scene of their accident in fright, thereby increasing the injuries or becoming lost and unavailable for veterinary care. DO NOT leave your cat unattended for one second. If necessary ask a bystander to telephone your veterinarian, or carry your animal with you to the telephone. (But before moving them, check for possible fractures or spinal cord damage. See below.)

First, evaluate your cat for signs of shock. A fracture or large cut can be spectacular and frightening, but this matter takes secondary consideration. If signs of shock are present,

Look For Signs Of Shock

171

be sure your cat gets professional veterinary care at once.

External And Internal Bleeding
A small amount of blood can appear to be more than it is. Try to determine the source of the blood loss. When you find the site, you will often find that the original bleeding has stopped. If there is a great deal of bleeding from the wound, apply a makeshift pressure bandage or direct pressure to it (see page 170). Persistent bleeding from the nose and/or mouth requires immediate veterinary care, as does blood in the urine or signs that indicate internal bleeding and/or injury (shock, abdominal pain, difficult breathing).

Broken Bones
A veterinarian should be consulted if you think your cat has a fractured limb, but the fracture itself may not be an emergency if the cat is doing well otherwise (see page 143). *Paralysis or partial paralysis may indicate spinal cord damage* and requires that you keep the vertebral column as immobile as possible from the time of the accident until you

arrive at the veterinary hospital (see page 145). A small box or cat carrier is the best means to carry a severely injured cat. If you can't determine the extent of the injury or do not have a make-shift carrier available, try carrying the cat as illustrated.

Internal Injuries
If you find that your cat seems essentially normal following an accident, you may not need to see a veterinarian. You should be aware, however, that certain major internal injuries may not be apparent for several hours (sometimes days) following such trauma.

Diaphragmatic Hernia
A *diaphragmatic hernia* results when a tear in the diaphragm allows abdominal organs to move through it into the chest. If the tear occurs at the time of an accident, but the actual hernia does not (or is mild), you may not see any signs. When the abdominal organs herniate (or a small hernia gets worse) strained respiration ensues. Lack of appetite, difficulty swallowing or vomiting may be seen. If you try to hear the heart sounds, they may be absent or muffled. If a large portion of the abdominal organs have moved into the

172

chest, you may notice a "tucked up" abdomen. Watch for signs indicating possible diaphragmatic hernia for several weeks following any severe accident.

Be sure to watch for signs of normal urination following incidents involving abdominal trauma, such as that suffered when a cat is hit by a car. Cats with ruptured bladders may act normally at first then later develop abdominal pain. Their abdomens may be very tender when examined. If urination is completely absent or blood-stained or if normal looking urine is passed with some difficulty, suspect a ruptured bladder, which is a surgical emergency.

Ruptured Bladder

If your cat is not examined by a veterinarian following an accident be sure to give them a thorough physical examination yourself, and watch them closely for signs of shock for twenty-four hours (keep them indoors). Don't forget to examine the abdomen thoroughly by palpation. If your cat shows signs of pain such as *tensing* (contracting) the abdominal muscles more than usual or crying out, or if the abdomen feels unusual to you (too few, too many, or unusually shaped masses present), be sure to arrange for an examination by a veterinarian.

Artificial Respiration

Any occasion in which you have to resort to artificial respiration is an emergency (except perhaps in a newborn kitten that is slow to start breathing).

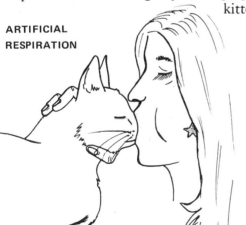

ARTIFICIAL RESPIRATION

Don't spend all your time trying to revive the cat on the spot. As soon as your veterinarian is contacted, head for the clinic while continuing attempts at resuscitation. Artificial respiration serves no purpose in an already dead

173

animal. Place your ear on the unconscious cat's chest and listen for a heart beat; feel for a pulse (see page 37). If no

Signs Of Death pulse or heart beat is detectable and the pupils are dilated and non-responsive to light, it is probable that death has already occurred and that your first aid will be useless.

To administer artificial respiration, open the mouth, pull out the tongue and look as far back into the pharynx as possible for any obstructions that may be present. If you can't see anything, it is a good idea to feel for obstructions with your fingers. Wipe away excessive mucous or blood in the pharynx that might interfere with air flow. Then close the cat's mouth. Inhale. Holding the cat's mouth closed, place your mouth over their nose (cover it completely) and exhale in an attempt to force the exhaled air through the cat's nose into the chest. (It may be easier to do if you allow your mouth to cover the whole muzzle.) Then watch for the chest to expand as you blow. After inflating the lungs in this manner, remove your mouth to allow the chest to return to its original (deflated) position. Repeat the inflation-deflation cycle about six times per minute as long as necessary.

External Heart Massage

External heart massage is used in an attempt to maintain circulation when cardiac arrest has occurred. If you cannot feel a pulse or heart beat in an unconscious and non-breathing cat, you may try external cardiac massage. Heart arrest automatically follows respiratory arrest, or when heart arrest occurs first, breathing soon stops. Therefore, *cardiac massage must be combined with artificial respiration if any benefit is to be gained.* Irreversible damage to the brain is said to occur after three minutes without oxygen. This implies that heart massage must be started within three to five minutes following cardiac arrest to be of benefit.

Place the cat on its right side on a firm surface. Place the fingers of one hand on each side of the chest over the area of the heart and compress it *firmly*. (Don't worry too much about damage to the chest—getting effective circulation is more important.) Then completely release the pressure. This cycle should be repeated about seventy times per minute.

174

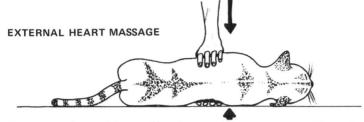

EXTERNAL HEART MASSAGE

You can also achieve effective cardiac massage with a single hand wrapped around the chest. If you are being effective you should be able to feel a pulse (see page 37) with each massage.

While attempts to restart the heart are being made, try to get the animal to a veterinarian. Don't expect the animal to revive during your attempts at resuscitation before obtaining veterinary services. If consciousness resumes, however, keep the cat warm and quiet and proceed to a veterinary hospital where observation can continue.

Convulsions

Convulsions (seizures) include a wide variety of signs consisting primarily of abnormal behavior and/or abnormal body movements. The most easily recognized signs are *loss* (or disturbance) *of consciousness, loss of motor control,* and *involuntary urination* and/or *defecation.* Convulsions fall into two main catagories in terms of whether or not they are emergencies:

1. The single convulsion which lasts for a minute or two and does not recur for at least twenty-four hours.

2. Repeated or continuous convulsions.

Consulsions in the second catagory require immediate veterinary attention. Cats with convulsions in the first category should be examined by a veterinarian, but may not require emergency care.

The most important thing for you to do if your cat is having a convulsion is to provide gentle restraint so they won't injure themselves. One of the best ways is to place a light blanket or towel over the cat. It's not a good idea to place your hand on the cat or in or near their mouth unless you are willing to risk serious scratches or bites. Airway occlusion due to the tongue rarely occurs. While one person

Restraint Is Important

175

restrains the cat, another can try to reach a veterinarian. Seizures in the first catagory are often passed by the time you get in touch with a veterinarian.

Poisoning

Emergency situations involving convulsions occur commonly following poisonings. Cats are extremely sensitive to the effects of many chemicals used commonly in the house and garden, but because of their habits they are not often seen to ingest the poisonous substance. Instead an owner often only becomes aware that poisoning has occurred after signs of toxicity, such as convulsions, develop. Try to prevent poisoning from common household products by reading their labels carefully and using them appropriately. Any product labeled hazardous for humans should be assumed to be toxic to your cat as well. Outdoors avoid the use of organophosphate and chlorinated hydrocarbon insecticides (see chart), snail baits, herbicides, fungicides and rodent poisons if there is even the slightest chance your cat may come into contact with them.

General Treatment Of Poisoning

1. If you see your cat ingest a toxic substance, induce vomiting unless the material is corrosive (strong acid, alkali or petroleum distillate, e.g., kerosene). The most reliable way to cause vomiting is to adminster about a teaspoonful of *hydrogen peroxide* by mouth. If vomiting does not occur within five to ten minutes, you can repeat the dose at least two more times. Another method you can try is to place about one-fourth teaspoonful of salt on the back of the cat's tongue. (If signs of poisoning are already apparent when you first see the animal, DO NOT try to cause vomition, but rush the cat to a veterinarian.) Following vomition (or if induction of vomiting is not indicated on chart below) give milk mixed with a raw egg at approximately one-fourth cup per ten pounds body weight.

2. If your cat gets a toxic substance on their skin, flush with large volumes of water while (or before) someone calls a veterinarian for further advice.

3. If convulsions occur, try to restrain the cat (see page 175).

4. Try to bring a sample of the suspected poison *in its original container* to the hospital.

Poison	Common Products Containing It	Immediate Treatment If Exposure Known	Signs Which May Develop Following Exposure
Ethylene glycol	Antifreeze	Induce vomiting and rush to veterinarian.	Immediate treatment necessary. DO NOT wait for signs to appear.
Organophosphate	Insecticides— coumaphos, dichlorvos, malathion, fenthion, ronnel.	On skin: wash with alkaline detergent and wait for signs to appear.	Salivation, small pupils, muscle tremors, vomiting, diarrhea, incoordination, convulsions.
Chlorinated hydrocarbons	Insecticides— methoxychlor, toxaphene, lindane, chlordane	On skin: wash with soap and water and wait for signs	Salivation, diarrhea, hyperexcitability, muscle twitches, convulsions.
Strychnine	Rodent poisons, malicious poisonings	Induce vomiting if signs not yet present.	Restlessness, incoordination, muscle tremors, convulsions.
Metaldehyde	Snail bait	Induce vomiting if signs not yet present.	Restlessness, incoordination, muscle tremors, vomiting, convulsions.
Salicylate (aspirin)	Aspirin	Avoid use; spontaneous consumption unlikely.	Weakness, lack of appetite, vomiting, fever, incoordination, convulsions.
Phenol (carbolic acid)	Household disinfectants and antiseptics, wood preservatives, fungicides, herbicides, photographic developer	On skin: wash with soap and water. Ingested: induce vomiting and wait for signs to appear.	Incoordination, muscle tremors, depression, unconsciousness.
Amphetamine	Diet and stimulant pills	Induce vomiting, wait for signs to appear.	Delirium, fever, dilated pupils, convulsions, shock, unconsciousness.
Arsenic	Ant poisons, herbicides, insecticides	Induce vomiting, and consult veterinarian immediately. No home treatment effective.	Vomiting, restlessness, abdominal pain, diarrhea (sometimes bloody).

Common Household Poisons and Their Treatment

177

Thallium	Rodent poison	Consult veterinarian, no effective home remedy.	Signs vary.
Warfarin	Rodent poison	Consult veterinarian, no effective home remedy. Single dose may not cause signs.	Hemorrhage-mainly internal. Pale mucous membranes, weakness.
Alkali	Cleaning preparations, grease dissolvers, drain opener (sodium, potassium, ammonium hydroxide)	On skin: water and vinegar rinse. Ingested: vinegar by mouth.	
Acids	Car batteries, some metal cleaners	On skin: flush with water, apply bicarbonate paste. Ingested: magnesium hydroxide antacid, egg white, sodium bicarbonate.	
Phosphorus	Strike anywhere matches (safety matches nontoxic), rat poisons, fireworks	Induce vomiting	Vomiting, diarrhea, abdominal pain, collapse.

Poisonous Plants

The list of potentially dangerous house and garden plants is very long. The best rule to follow is to watch your cat carefully and correct them if they chew on plants. Some of the more common poisonous plants are:

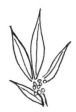

Plant	Poisonous Parts
Castor bean	Seeds and foliage
Oleander	All parts
Monkshood	All parts
Philodendron	Leaves
Autumn crocus	All parts
English Ivy	Leaves, berries
Lily of the Valley	Leaves, flowers
Daphne	Bark, leaves, flowers

178

Plant	Poisonous Parts
Larkspur	Young plants, seeds
Foxglove	Leaves
Golden chain	Leaves, seeds
Daffodil	Bulbs

Dumbcane *(Diffenbachia)*, a common houseplant, causes irritation of the mouth, laryngitis, and temporary paralysis of the vocal cords when eaten.

Snakebite

Although cases of snakebite in cats are rare, you should be aware of the first aid necessary in order to try to prevent death if your cat should be bitten by a snake. Prompt action by you and your veterinarian is necessary. Bites of poisonous snakes cause severe pain, so a bitten animal will often become excited and run. You should attempt to prevent this response, if at all possible, since exercise helps spread the venom. Immobilize the cat as soon as possible (place them in a small box or cat carrier).

If the bite is on an extremity, apply a flat tourniquet between the body and the wound (nearest the wound). The tourniquet should be loose enough to barely slip one finger under, and it *should not* be fully loosened until the bite is treated by a veterinarian or until two hours have passed. (This type of application allows some oxygen to reach the tissues beyond the tourniquet.) If possible keep a bitten limb on a level horizontal with the heart (i.e., lay the cat on their side). Then make linear incisions (not x-shaped) over the fang wounds and apply suction (preferably not by mouth but with a suction cup). (For coral snake bites, *immediately* apply a tight tourniquet and *quickly* cut away a wide area of tissue surrounding and including the fang wounds.)

Get your cat to a veterinarian as soon as possible. Since a cat in pain is difficult at best to handle, the best first aid may be only to apply a tight tourniquet and acquire veterinary aid within fifteen minutes. The veterinarian will administer antivenin, antibiotics and pain relievers, and can administer other medical treatment as necessary. It may be

179

necessary to remove a large portion of the wound surgically. Even if this is not done, snake bites often cause large portions of skin to die and slough, leaving a large wound which must be treated. Plan on your cat being hospitalized for a minimum of twenty-four to forty-eight hours if snakebite occurs.

Fishhooks in Skin

Fishhooks become embedded easily as foreign bodies in the skin. Once the barb has passed under the skin, a hook will not fall out on its own. The only way to remove it is to push the barb through the skin. Once through, cut the curved part of the hook just below the barb and pull the rest of the hook back out through the original hole. Often this procedure is too painful to be accomplished without anesthesia so don't be surprised if you need the help of a veterinarian. Veterinary services are needed to administer appropriate antibiotics as well; unless the hook was *extremely* clean, this type of wound is likely to become infected.

Where
To
Cut

Porcupine Quills in Skin

The important thing to remember about a procupine quill in the skin is to remove the *whole* thing. Grasp the quill with a pair of pliers near the point where it disappears into the skin; then, with a quick tug, pull it out. If the quill breaks off as you try to remove it or if some of the quills have broken off before you had a chance to try to remove them, you may need a veterinarian's help. DO NOT ignore pieces of quill you cannot pull from the skin. They can migrate long distances (sometimes into bone) carrying sources of infection with them. And remember to check for quills inside the mouth as well as in the body surface.

Insect Bite or Sting

Owners usually become aware of insect bites or stings long after they have happened. Usually a large swelling of the muzzle tissue is noticed with no particular evidence of pain. Other times hives (bumps in the skin) appear. These are allergic reactions to the bite or sting. If there is no fever and

180

if the cat acts normally (even though abnormal in appearance), no treatment is usually necessary, but pull out the stinger if you see it. Swelling should go away within about forty-eight hours. If you catch the bite early, or if signs such as difficulty breathing or extreme swelling begin to occur, consult a veterinarian. Corticosteroids may be administered to prevent signs or further progression of signs already apparent.

Burns

Burns may be thermal, chemical or electrical (electric shock). The severity of *thermal* (heat) burns in cats may be *Thermal* underestimated because their appearance differs considerably *Burns* from those in man. Blisters characteristic of superficial burns in humans may not form in the burned skin of a cat. Instead the hair remains firmly attached in a superficial burn. If you pull on the hair in the area of a burn and it comes out easily, the burn is deeper and more serious.

Immediate treatment of thermal burns consists of applying cold water or ice compresses for twenty minutes. A soothing antibacterial medication can then be applied. Deep burns or burns convering large areas need emergency veterinary care. Because of the difficulty in evaluating the severity of burns in cat skin immediately after their occurrence, it is a good idea to have all burns examined by a veterinarian within twenty-four hours.

Electrical burns often occur in young cats who bite into electric cords while playing. They can cause severe damage to *Electrical* the skin of the mouth and *pulmonary edema* (fluid in the *Burns* lungs). Cats sustaining such burns should be thoroughly *(Electric* examined by a veterinarian as soon as you become aware of *Shock)* the injury. If difficult breathing or coughing occurs, pulmonary edema may be present. In severe cases the tongue and gums may look bluish. If you find your cat unconscious and not breathing after electric shock, administer artificial respiration (see page 173). If general signs do not develop after electric shock, mouth tissue damaged by the burn often dies and sloughs several days later and needs veterinary attention.

181

Chemical
Burns
For information on chemical burns, see *acids* and *alkali* in the chart of common household poisons page 178.

Heat Stress (Heat Stroke)

Heat stress occurs most often in animals that have been confined to a car (or other enclosure) with inadequate ventilation on a warm day. Temperatures inside a parked, poorly ventilated car can rapidly reach over one hundred degrees F on a relatively mild seventy-five to eighty degree day. Heat stress can also occur in animals suddenly transported to a hot climate to which they have not been previously acclimatized. Young cats, fat cats and older cats are more subject to heat stress than others.

Signs Of
Heat Stress
Signs of heat stress are panting, increased pulse rate, congested mucous membranes (reddened gums), *and an anxious or staring expression.* Vomiting may occur. Stupor and unconsciousness may follow if the stress is allowed to continue long enough. Rectal temperatures are elevated (106 to 109 degrees F). Immediate treatment by immersion in cold water is necessary. If you cannot immerse the cat, spray them with cold water. Massage the skin and flex and extend the legs to return blood from the peripheral circulation. Then get your cat to a veterinary hospital where treatment can be continued.

Cats sustaining heat stress should always be examined by a veterinarian, but if this is impossible, take their temperature frequently over a twenty-four hour period because elevation of the rectal temperature often recurs after the initial drop and first signs of improvement. It has been suggested that if the rectal temperature has not reached 103 degrees F in ten to fifteen minutes after starting treatment, a cold water enema should be given. Following this treatment, however, the rectal temperature is no longer accurate.

You Can
Prevent
Heat Stress
Prevent heat stroke by carrying water with you when you travel on hot days and by giving your cat small amounts frequently. Wet towels placed directly over your cat or over their carrier will provide cooling by evaporation. Open car windows when a cat is left inside, or better yet, don't leave the animal in the car.

182

Eclampsia (Puerperal Tetany, Milk Fever)

Eclampsia *(puerperal tetany)* usually occurs in mother cats within two or three weeks after delivery, although it can occur before delivery. Though the exact cause is unknown, it is due to a defect in calcium metabolism which results in an abnormally low blood calcium level. Although it occurs infrequently in cats, heavily lactating females with large litters seem predisposed to the disease.

The first signs are often restlessness, crying and rapid breathing. Spontaneous recovery may result, or the signs may progress to stiffness and muscle spasms, incoordination, recumbency, convulsions and fever. *Progressive tetany is an emergency* which must be treated by a veterinarian. Calcium preparations are given intravenously. Kittens are removed from nursing for at least twenty-four hours. Sometimes they may be returned to restricted nursing later, but this must be supplemented by hand feeding. Kittens old enough to eat solid food are weaned. Calcium-phosphorus-vitamin D supplements are often prescribed for queens who must continue restricted nursing.

Certain females seem predisposed to milk fever and it may be advisable not to rebreed these females. A ration adequate in calcium, phosphorus and vitamin D should be fed throughout pregnancy. Some veterinarians, however, feel that oversupplementation may help induce milk fever. Therefore supplementation during pregnancy should be with balanced vitamin-mineral preparations used cautiously. Discuss this problem in detail with your veterinarian.

Geriatric Medicine
(Care as Your Cat Ages)

General Information

The life expectancy of the cat varies considerably between individuals and with the kind of health care received throughout their life. Most well-cared-for cats can be expected to live between ten and fifteen years and many reach the age of twenty. A few cats have even been reported to have lived as long as thirty years.

Old Cats May Not Adjust Well To Changes — In general the older cat is less adaptable to stress. Sudden changes in diet, routine or environment are probably best avoided if they have not been part of the cat's routine in the past. Many old cats do not adapt well to hospitalization and therefore need special care when ill. Good veterinarians are aware of this and provide special attention or make special arrangements for the care of such older animals.

Geriatric Diet — If you have been feeding your cat a well-balanced diet throughout their life, few if any changes will be needed in old age unless special health conditions develop. Special diets need to be provided for older cats with degenerative changes of major organs such as the kidneys. Many other times the addition of a balanced vitamin-mineral supplement to the normal diet is sufficient to meet any special needs imposed by the aging process. Sometimes strong smelling foods, such as those containing fish or fish oil, stimulate a lagging appetite which is the result of decreased ability to smell or taste. Since each cat is an individual and ages as an individual, the need for a special diet should be discussed with a veterinarian familiar with your aging cat before any major dietary changes are made.

Geriatric Exercise — Most cats continue to exercise and play to the degree they have most of their lives well into old age. Only rarely is there a reason to restrict an older cat's activity, and the best rule to follow is to allow your cat to exercise as they choose. Watch carefully for sudden changes in activity; they can indicate illness.

Some conditions which are likely to develop in cats with age are covered in this section. Not all are disabling or progressive and most, if recognized early, can be treated at

184

least palliatively. To use this section for diagnosing signs, refer to the Index of Signs on page 113 as well as to the General Index.

Lens Sclerosis

The formation of new fibers in the lens of the cat's eye continues throughout life. As new fibers are formed the older ones are compressed and pushed toward the center of the lens. The lens also loses water as it ages, a factor contributing to increased density as well. This process is called *nuclear sclerosis* and should be recognized as a normal part of the aging of the cat's eye. It results in a bluish or greyish-white haze in the part of the lens which can be seen through the pupil. It *does not* normally interfere with vision and does not need treatment. This condition is often erroneously referred to as *cataracts* (lens opacities which interfere with light transmission to the retina). In truth, senile cataracts, which usually appear very white and dense and which interfere with vision, occur much less commonly.

If your cat does develop cataracts as an aged (or sometimes young) animal and loss of vision occurs, there are surgical procedures which can be used to remove the opacity and restore vision. This surgery is not performed routinely, however, because cataracts are relatively uncommon and most cats seem to adjust completely to a gradual loss of vision.

Deafness

Gradual loss of hearing occurs as cats age, but not as frequently as in older dogs. The anatomical changes responsible for hearing loss are not well established and treatment is not possible. Inattentiveness or unresponsiveness to calling is often one of the first signs of hearing loss. A crude test for hearing ability is to stand behind the cat and make a sudden sound, such as a whistle, hand clap or sharp call. Most cats will cock their ears toward the sound or turn their heads. Hands clapped near the ear (but not near or in front of the eyes) may cause both eyes to blink in response to the sound.

185

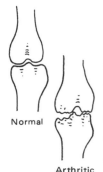

Normal

Arthritic

Osteoarthritis (Arthritis)

Osteoarthritis is a joint disease in which the *cartilages* (fibrous caps) covering the articular surfaces of the bones degenerate and bony proliferation (excesss bone growth) occurs. This condition usually results in pain and lameness of the involved joints. It may occur in single joints of young animals with congenital joint defects or following any kind of joint trauma. When it occurs as an aging change it affects several joints, although lameness may not be apparent in all those affected. The lameness present with arthritis is often most severe on arising and improves with exercise. If you gently move the affected joints you may hear or feel *crepitus* (bone grating against bone). X-ray films will show the affected joints and the severity of bone changes. Although you may not become aware of the disease until signs occur, the changes characteristic of arthritis have usually been occurring over a long prior period.

There is no effective means of arresting the progression of osteoarthritis in older cats so treatment is usually symptomatic, directed at relieving any significant pain. Unfortunately most drugs useful for the symptomatic relief of arthritis in people, dogs and other animals are toxic to cats. One of the safest drugs for people or dogs, aspirin, can cause severe signs of illness in cats and must only be used with care under the direction of a veterinarian. Fortunately few cats with osteoarthritis show discomfort and intermittent lameness or lameness that is only present on arising usually needs no treatment. Weight reduction often significantly improves lameness in obese cats with arthritis. If signs of pain are significant, the aid of a veterinarian can be of help in providing relief.

Tumors (Neoplasms, Cancer)

A *tumor* is an abnormal growth of tissue *(neoplasm* means new growth). *Benign tumors* are those which are likely to remain at the site of their original growth. *Malignant tumors* (cancer) are neoplastic growths which invade surrounding tissue and travel via blood vessels or lymph channels to other body sites where they start to grow anew.

186

Although cats as a breed have a comparatively high incidence of cancer (see page 165), the likelihood of any tumor occurring increases with age.

Many tumors occur internally where you would not likely be aware of them until they have grown quite large. You should, however, watch carefully for growths in the mouth and on the outside of your cat's body. On females it is wise to check each mammary gland periodically (e.g., once a month) for new growths. If you find a tumor in a young or aged cat, it is always best to discuss its removal with a veterinarian. If you don't feel that you can see a veterinarian, watch the tumor carefully for growth. Some malignant tumors *metastasize* (spread) while the original tumor is still very small.

Constipation

Difficult or infrequent passage of stools (constipation) is one of the more common but usually not serious problems of older cats. Aging changes often result in loss of muscle tone which when combined with a suboptimal diet or changes in the digestive process result in recurrent constipation. Home remedies for constipation discussed on page 151 can be used to treat constipation in older cats. Don't rely on any methods repeatedly except the dietary changes mentioned unless your veterinarian directs you to do so after giving your cat a clean bill of health.

Kidney Disease

Many older cats have decreased kidney function due to aging changes and/or urinary tract disease processes which have gone undetected earlier in life. Because the kidneys have a large amount of tissue reserve, signs attributable to progressive kidney disease are often not apparent without laboratory tests until damage is severe and often irreversible.

Increased water drinking accompanied by increased volume of urination are often signs of kidney disease. As the kidneys degenerate, less functioning tissue is available to excrete the same amount of wastes produced by the body as when the kidneys were healthy. In an effort to maintain a

187

normal physiological state, a larger volume of urine in which the wastes are less concentrated must be excreted and the cat must drink more water daily. The need to excrete large volumes of urine will sometimes cause an old cat without a litter box and without convenient access to the outside to urinate in the house. This cat has not "forgotten their housetraining" or "grown senile;" the volume of urine is just too great to be held. The only way to remedy this situation is to provide a litter pan indoors or to provide more easy access to the outdoors. Restricting water availability will not help, but can actually make the cat sick, since it interferes with waste excretion.

When a cat cannot compensate for failing kidneys, vomiting, lack of appetite and weight loss are other signs that may develop. The teeth may be unsightly and the breath abnormally odorous (ammonia-like). If you feel the kidneys they may feel abnormally small (most common in older cats) or abnormally large. If your cat has any signs of failing kidneys consult your veterinarian immediately. Other diseases (e.g., *diabetes mellitus*) may have similar signs and diagnosis requires laboratory tests including urinalysis and blood tests. Your veterinarian will try to find out if the disease process can be arrested and advise you on care which can prolong your cat's comfortable life in spite of diseased kidneys.

Heart Disease

Heart disease is not common in cats of any age. When heart disease occurs, however, it is of several types, just as there are several types which occur in people and in dogs. Heart disease in cats presents frequently as *congestive heart failure* seen in older cats when the heart, which has progressively become more inefficient as a blood pump, is no longer able to supply the needs of the body tissues (*heart failure*). It is important to understand that heart disease (of many types) can be present long before actual failure occurs. Heart disease generally progresses through several stages where it can be treated and the signs ameliorated before heart failure requiring emergency treatment or resulting in death

188

occurs.

A *murmur* caused by abnormal turbulence of blood in a diseased heart may be the first sign of heart disease. Your veterinarian may mention a murmur's presence at the time of your cat's yearly physical exam and booster shots. Or you may hear a murmur as a "shh" sound interposed between the normal lub-dup sounds of the heart beat when you are examining your cat. If the murmur is intense enough you may even be able to feel it through the chest wall as the heart beats. The presence of a murmur in any age cat is not necessarily something to be alarmed about, but it is something that requires examination by a veterinarian. They may suggest chest x-rays, an electrocardiogram, a complete blood count and other tests. *Heart Murmurs*

In cases where you cannot detect a murmur or a murmur is not present you may not notice any changes until uncompensated heart failure occurs. At this time there may be difficult breathing (due to fluid accumulation in the lungs and chest); the heart rate becomes extremely rapid and the cat is reluctant to move or eat. Death soon follows if treatment is not intitiated. *Signs Of Heart Failure*

Treatment of heart disease in the older cat is generally directed at improving circulatory function, since the aging process cannot be arrested. Medical treatment includes drugs which dilate the airways, *digitalis*-like drugs to increase the strength of heart contraction and *diuretics* to help control sodium and water retention that accompany heart failure. If drug treatment is successful you will be asked to continue it at home and to provide a diet of foods low in sodium if possible. Continued home treatment for heart disease in the older animal can be relatively easy and the benefits include a longer, more comfortable and more active life for the cat.

Euthanasia

It would be nice if all old pets died peacefully in their sleep with no previous signs of illness. This doesn't always happen, though, and sometimes you must decide whether to end your cat's life or allow a progressive or painful disease to continue. This is never an easy decision. A mutually close and trusting relationship with a veterinarian established when your cat is still young may help if you ever have to face this problem. A veterinarian familiar with your cat's medical history can tell you when a condition is irreversible and progressive and can give you an opinion as to when that condition is truly a burden for your cat.

It is unfair to you, your pet, and the veterinarian to take an animal to a new veterinarian and request euthanasia. A veterinarian not familiar with your cat may perform euthanasia because you requested it when the condition was actually treatable. A veterinarian unfamiliar with you may refuse this heart-rending act because your cat seems healthy not knowing that continuing to live with the cat is a burden for you Most veterinarians enter the profession to make animals well, not to kill them. Too often I see people who react emotionally without knowing the facts, and insist that their pet be "put to sleep" for a condition which can be treated and with which their cat can live happily. In other cases euthanasia is requested because a new pet is cheaper than treatment. The joy of life outweighs minor discomforts for most people, and I believe (perhaps too anthropomorphically) for most pets as well. The monetary value of a pet's life, I suppose, depends on each individual's philosophy. A veterinarian you know well and who knows your pet can present the medical facts about a sick or aged pet openly for you to use in making your final decision. If you decide you just don't want a healthy animal any more, give it to a friend that does want it, or take it to a shelter or pound where humane euthansia is performed if you find it impossible to provide the animal with a new and loving home.

When you and your veterinarian agree about ending the life of a pet, you need not worry about discomfort. Euthansia in most veterinary hospitals is performed by the intravenous injection of an overdose of an anesthetic drug. Death is both rapid and painless.

Home Medical Care

Nursing at Home
Drug Information

Your Cat's Medical Record

Date	Temperature	Stool	Urine	Miscellaneous — include here medication, times given, times wounds cleaned, unusual signs, changes, etc.

Xerox this page to use for record keeping while nursing your pet at home.

Home Medical Care
Nursing at Home

Although the average cat has few illnesses requiring prolonged hospitalization during their lifetime, many minor illnesses can become severe if proper home care is not provided. Most veterinarians are anxious to have your cat recover at home if they think you can provide adequate nursing. It's also a lot cheaper and will draw you close to your animal. This section is designed to give you the information you need for basic home nursing. If you become familiar with its contents you should be able to treat most minor illnesses diagnosed by your veterinarian at home. In cases where there are no alternatives to hospitalization, familiarity with basic nursing techniques should allow the hospital stay to be shortened and more of the convalescence to occur at home.

Record Keeping

If your cat has a serious illness, regular and accurate record keeping is invaluable in helping your veterinarian help you treat your cat at home. Take your cat's temperature at least once daily (preferably around the same time) and record the value. Record how much your cat eats and drinks, how often they urinate and the type of bowel movements they pass. This, of course, requires that your cat be kept indoors and a litter box provided. In some instances it is best to confine the recovering cat to one room or a small area; other times the cat can be allowed to wander freely around the house. Your veterinarian can help you decide on the best kind of confinement. In no instance, however, should a sick cat be allowed to roam freely unsupervised outdoors. Sick cats frequently disappear only to be found later in much worse condition than when they left, or never to return at all. Additional helpful information to keep in your records includes an indication of the times and amounts of medication given and a record of any unusual signs (e.g., vomiting) which develop or any other change in condition. Take these records with you whenever you visit the veterinarian. In addition, scanning the progress of your animal's recovery can teach you more about how the body heals itself.

Temperature

Use a rectal thermometer to take your cat's temperature. An oral thermometer can be used in a pinch, but the bulb is more likely to break off. Before inserting the thermometer into the rectum, shake the mercury column down below ninety-nine degrees F and lubricate the tip of it with any non-toxic greasy substance (petroleum jelly, lubricant jelly, vegetable oil). Place your cat on a table or other level platform; hold your cat's tail up with one hand, and insert the thermometer into the rectum with a firm, gentle push. You may feel some resistance to the thermometer just after you pass through the anus; this is due to the cat's strong internal anal sphincter muscle. When you encounter this resistance

RESTRAINT WHILE TAKING A CAT'S TEMPERATURE

194

just continue to push gently but firmly until the muscle relaxes and allows the thermometer to pass, or rotate the thermometer gently. This is most easily done with the cat standing, but can be done while they sit or lie down. How far you need to insert the thermometer to get an accurate rectal temperature depends on the size of the cat—an inch to and inch and one-half is usually sufficient. If you feel the thermometer go into a fecal mass when you insert it, try again. The thermometer should be left two or three minutes although many thermometers will register an accurate temperature in about one minute. (Helpful information if you have an uncooperative cat!)

THERMOMETER

To read the thermometer, roll it back and forth between your fingers until you can see the thin mercury column inside. The point where the column stops is the temperature. Each large mark indicates one degree, each small mark two-tenths of a degree.

Pulse, Heart Rate

For how to take your cat's pulse and measure the heart rate see page 37.

How to Pill Your Cat

The only way to be sure your cat has really swallowed medication in pill, capsule or tablet form is to administer it in the following way: Place your cat on a table or other similar platform and get them to sit or stand relatively quietly. Grasp the pill between the thumb and forefinger of one hand so you have it ready to administer. Then place the opposite hand over the top of your cat's head, thumb and index finger near the corners of the mouth as illustrated on page 28 and tilt the head backwards until the nose points toward the ceiling. Press against the cat's lips with your index finger and

195

thumb to open the mouth and use the third finger of your pill-containing hand to hold the lower jaw open. Then quickly drop or place the pill over the back of the cat's tongue. (With practice, you can give the pill a quick and gentle shove with your index finger to send it on its way down the throat.) Then immediately allow the cat's mouth to close and hold it tightly closed until the pill is swallowed. (To be successful be sure to keep the cat's nose pointed upward during the whole procedure.) It is extremely important to perform these maneuvers quickly and smoothly if pilling is to be successful. If you spend too long in preparation, an uncooperative cat has mustered their full counterforces by the time you actually attempt to give the drug and you are destined for failure. Although it may seem difficult at first, with a little practice giving medication in solid form becomes very easy in all but the fiercest cats. In preparation for the day when you may have to nurse your cat at home, it is a good idea to go through the motions of administering medication to develop skill while your cat is still young, cooperative and healthy. You can use a piece of dry kibble as a practice pill.

PUSHING THE PILL DOWN

Problems most often occur when the pill is not placed or dropped properly over the base of the tongue. If you drop it off center or not far enough back, the cat will spit it out or bite into it. If this happens and the cat is still cooperative, try again. Many times when this occurs the cat tastes the medication and begins to drool profusely. This is no cause for

196

concern, but usually requires that you wait a few minutes before trying to administer the medication again. Buttering uncoated tablets helps with this problem, and is also useful if pills don't seem slippery enough or seem a little on the large side. If you find it absolutely impossible to give solid medication in the manner described you can try crushing a tablet or pill or emptying the contents of a capsule and mixing the drug thoroughly with a small portion of meat or some other favorite food. Sometimes the medicine can be mixed with water and administered as a liquid. Most medicines taste so bad that a sick cat will not take them voluntarily in food or liquid. So if it can be avoided, do not use these methods of administration. You can never be sure that your cat has taken all the medicine when it is administered in food. If you grind an *enteric-coated* (coated to be absorbed in the intestine) tablet or empty the contents of a capsule into food, you may be preventing normal absorption of the drug from the gut. Coverings are often designed to remain intact until the drugs reaches the part of the gut where it is best and most safely absorbed.

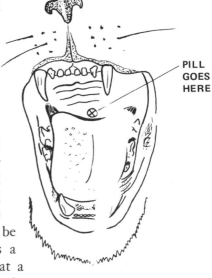

PILL
GOES
HERE

Liquid Medication

The simplest way to give your cat liquid medication is to squirt it into the back of the mouth using an eyedropper or syringe (hypodermic or infant ear type). For most liquid medicines your veterinarian will automatically provide you with the tool necessary to administer the medication; if they do not, request them to and also request a demonstration of its use. To administer a liquid, grasp the head as if you were going to give a pill (see page 196), then slip the dropper between the cat's rear teeth and squirt in the liquid, or if the cat opens their mouth far enough, just squirt the liquid onto the back of the tongue. Keep the cat's nose pointed upward while they swallow the liquid. Otherwise they will tend to shake their head and spit out the medicine. Give only small amounts at a time (¼ teaspoonful, 1 cc) and allow swallowing to occur between each portion to avoid causing the cat to choke or inhale the liquid.

Force Feeding

Since lack of appetite (*anorexia*) accompanies many feline illnesses, coaxing or force feeding is often necessary to insure that sufficient calories and nutrients are consumed and to maintain the nutritional health necessary to the vital functions and repair of injured or diseased tissues. The effects of one day (or even more in a well-fleshed adult) without food, of course, are not irreversible, but prolonged refusal to eat forces the cat's body to draw upon its own vital tissues to obtain the calories necessary for vital function. If this process is allowed to continue for too long it can itself result in death, when the original disease would not have. Water is also very important to your cat's health and recovery, since dehydration begins as soon as water intake does not meet daily water need. (For more about dehydration see page 110). Water can be administered by the techniques used for force feeding of liquids, and since most foods used for force feeding contain a high proportion of water, hand administration of food helps meet the cat's daily water need. Use the following information about hand feeding whenever your veterinarian suggests that it is necessary and to help stabilize a sick cat's condition until veterinary help can be obtained. Do not, though, use hand feeding in lieu of a diagnosis; unless proper treatment is given, hand feeding alone cannot usually bring a cat back to health.

Liquid diets can be force fed to a sick cat in the same way liquid medication is given (see page 197). It is easier to feed solid or semi-solid diets by using your finger or a tongue

198

depressor (available in drugstores) to wipe the food onto the roof of your cat's mouth. (Grasp the cat's head as if giving a pill. Instead, insert your finger or the tongue depressor full of food and wipe it against the roof of the mouth.) Solid food can also be given rolled into small pellets like pills.

FEEDING WITH A SYRINGE

Good foods for temporary hand feeding of sick cats are strained baby foods. Strained egg yolk is best because of its high calorie content and high digestibility, but if your cat finds meat flavors more palatable, you can use strained chicken or turkey, lamb or beef baby foods, adding two egg yolks per three ounce jar (high protein, high calorie diet) or one tablespoon corn oil and one tablespoon corn syrup per three ounce jar (high fat, high calorie diet) or a combination of egg yolks, oil and/or corn syrup. Corn syrup and corn oil may also be added to egg baby foods to liquify them while increasing the calorie and carbohydrate content. Feed an adult cat at least two jars of plain strained egg yolk or one jar of baby food or egg yolk mixture daily. Regular cat foods can also be used for hand feeding; just remember to take the time to feed enough to supply your sick cat's daily calorie needs (twenty-five to thirty Calories per pound daily). If necessary your veterinarian can supply you with special dietary supplements designed specifically for hand-feeding sick cats. In addition to foods you should provide a balanced vitamin-mineral supplement as recommended by your veterinarian while your cat is sick—to meet their daily vitamin-mineral needs and any increased requirements caused by their illness.

Feed no more than one to two tablespoonsful (one-half to one ounce) food or liquid per pound body weight at each feeding, or vomiting is likely to occur. Maintain your cat's proper hydration by measuring their water intake and supplementing it by hand as necessary to provide about one and one-half tablespoonsful (three-fourths ounce) water per pound daily. (You can use milk if it doesn't cause diarrhea.)

199

Don't forget that water or other liquids mixed with foods to liquify them for force feeding contributes to meeting the cat's daily water need. If you find that your cat has signs of dehydration (see page 111) and is not improving as expected with hand feeding and your other treatment, be sure to consult your veterinarian. Sometimes only the specialized techniques available in veterinary hospitals can fill the needs of a sick cat.

Foods For Hand-Feeding Sick Cats

Food	Approximate Calorie Content
Strained egg yolk baby food	34/oz
Strained beef baby food	13/oz
Strained lamb baby food	16/oz
Strained turkey, chicken baby food	20/oz
Egg yolk (medium)	55
Whole egg (medium)	70
Whole milk	20/oz
Honey	60/tablespoonful
Corn syrup	55/tablespoonful
Corn oil	70/tablespoonful

For caloric content of commercial cat foods, see page 155.

Any of the above foods are suitable for hand-feeding sick cats unless the illness requires a special diet.

Use the table here and on page 154 to calculate the amounts you need to feed to meet your cat's daily protein, vitamin and mineral needs. Whole eggs should be cooked (e.g., soft boiled) before feeding or mixing with other foods. Add no more than one tablespoonful of corn syrup or honey and one tablespoonful of corn oil per three once jar of baby food unless otherwise directed by your veterinarian. Add milk, meat or chicken broth, or water as necessary to liquify the foods for hand administration and to help meet the sick cat's daily fluid requirement.

200

Eye Medication

USING EYE DROPS

Ophthalmic ointments are most easily applied into the conjunctival sac (see page 23). Use your thumb or forefinger to roll the lower eyelid gently downward and squeeze the ointment into the space exposed. Eye-drops should be instilled with the cat's nose tilted slightly upward. Use one hand to grasp the cat's muzzle and hold the lower lid open. Rest the base of the hand holding the dropper bottle above the eye to hold the upper lid open, then drop in the medication. Avoid touching the end of the ointment tube or dropper bottle to the eye to prevent contamination of the solution and injury to the eye.

Ear Treatment

When your cat's ears become inflamed (see page 132) a more thorough cleaning than you give them routinely is often necessary. In most cases inflamed ears should be examined and if cleaning is necessary it should be done by a veterinarian who will have the necessary tools for visualizing the ear canal and eardrum during and after cleaning. Also, if the ears seem painful when touched, anesthesia is usually necessary to make most cats hold still for a thorough and safe ear cleaning. Fortunately instances when ear cleaning in cats is necessary are infrequent.

Veterinarians use several methods for cleaning ears. In one method a rubber bulb syringe filled with warm water-antiseptic soap solution or a wax-dissolving solution is inserted into the ear canal and used to flush the fluid in and out of the ear. This is done several times and is followed by clear water or antiseptic rinses. The clean ear canal is dried with

BULB SYRINGE

cotton swabs and appropriate ear medication is instilled. Another method relies on cotton-tipped swabs and the use of an instrument called an *ear loop* to remove debris.

201

If you cannot take your cat to a veterinarian, the best way to clean their ears at home is to use a cotton swab in the

CLEANING
EARS

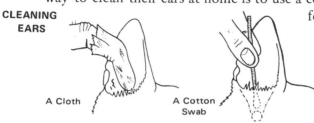

A Cloth   A Cotton
                    Swab

following manner. Grasp the end of the pinna (see page 24 and hold it straight up over the cat's head. Insert the swab into the ear canal parallel to the side of the head. You cannot damage the eardrum if you keep the swab vertical and parallel to the side of the head, but even if you don't, cats' ear canals are so narrow that it would be difficult to reach the eardrum with a cotton-tipped swab unless you were very rough and forceful. Use the swab to clean out debris before you start medication and once daily to remove old medication before instilling the new. Turn the swab gently and try to lift out debris rather than compacting it. Only a rare cat would allow you to clean the ears with the bulb syringe method without anesthesia. If you try it, use a warm solution, and flush the fluids in and out gently until all debris is removed. Then dry the canal gently with cotton-tipped swabs.

After your cat's ears are cleaned you will usually have to instill medication in them at least daily for one or two weeks. Most ear preparations have long nozzles which are placed into the ear canal. Liquids can be dropped into the canal. After

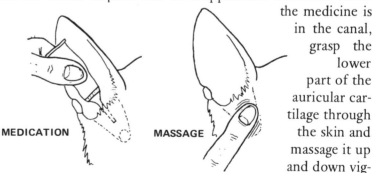

MEDICATION   MASSAGE

the medicine is in the canal, grasp the lower part of the auricular cartilage through the skin and massage it up and down vigorously. If you are doing it properly you will hear the medicine squishing around inside. This will spread the

202

medication down the length of the ear canal and is a very important part of nursing the ear properly. Once daily before instilling new medication it's a good idea to partially clean the ear to remove old medication and debris which accumulates. Use a cotton swab as described above or wrap your finger in a soft cloth or tissue and clean out the ear as far as your cloth-covered finger will reach.

Restraint

Unlike well-trained and frequently handled dogs most cats cannot be asked or commanded to sit, stand or lie quietly while unpleasant nursing procedures are performed. So to be successful in caring for your cat's health at home you need to learn the best ways to provide restraint when necessary to avoid injury to yourself and your cat and to allow the procedure to be carried out successfully. Cats vary greatly in their personalities and restraint must be tailored to the individual if you are to be successful. The best general rule to follow is to use the *minimum* amount of restraint necessary to achieve your goal. Never use two people when one is adequate and always try the gentlest method first, unless you know from experience with the cat that very firm restraint is necessary. All the basic home nursing procedures explained in this section are described as if performed by one person since most cats begin to struggle when firm restraint is applied, and since gentle control is the least stressful for the cat. If you find that these simple methods don't work for you, provide more firm control as necessary, but be sure to proceed firmly (not roughly) and deliberately or as the cat begins to object, you will lose your grip and may be scratched or bitten.

Never attempt treatment with the cat on the floor, the bed or in your lap unless the cat is very cooperative. To achieve the best success place them on a smooth-surfaced table or other level platform which allows you to stand next to it. The simplest way of restraint involves the use of one hand and/or arm leaving the other free for treatment. Light restraint includes placing one hand firmly over the cat's shoulders while they lie down or placing a hand in front of

203

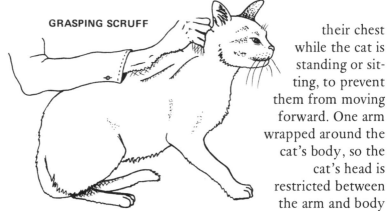

GRASPING SCRUFF

their chest while the cat is standing or sitting, to prevent them from moving forward. One arm wrapped around the cat's body, so the cat's head is restricted between the arm and body and so your hand can grasp their tail, provides good restraint for many procedures involving the rear legs and tail, as well as for taking a cat's temperature (see illustration page 194). For more control grasp the cat's *scruff* (skin at the base of the neck) tightly and firmly, or grasp the cat at the base of the skull and press firmly with your thumb and fingers. When using one of the these methods, you can, if necessary, rest the arm of your restraining hand down the cat's back to give you greater control.

If these simple holding methods fail and you have no one to help you, try rolling the cat in a towel or placing them in a pillow case. To give oral medication, allow the cat's head to protrude, then follow the directions given for administering solids or liquid medicines (see page 195). For other treatment just expose the area which needs care while leaving the rest of the cat covered. It is not always necessary to physically roll a cat in a towel. A towel just placed over an uncooperative cat often seems to calm them and

WRAPPED IN TOWEL

will sometimes allow you to grasp and treat an otherwise "impossible" patient. If at any time during these or the

204

following procedures the cat begins to pant or becomes

ASSISTANT HOLDING BOTH FORELEGS

visibly weaker, stop your restraint and allow the cat to regain their strength and composure before proceding. Weak cats overly stressed by fighting restraint may collapse.

Having two people working together makes nursing a very uncooperative cat much easier. When giving oral medication, your assistant can wrap their arms around the cat and grasp the front legs firmly, applying downward pressure to prevent them from reaching up while you handle the head and mouth. Or your assistant can wield the towel if you find that it is easier to give treatment with the cat partially covered. For other instances when firm restraint must be used your assistant can hold the cat in one of the following ways:

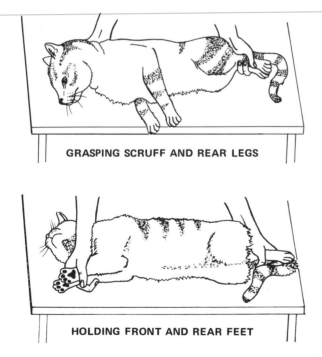

GRASPING SCRUFF AND REAR LEGS

HOLDING FRONT AND REAR FEET

205

Although most veterinarians rarely muzzle a cat and the times you would have to do it are few, a muzzle can be very helpful when treating a cat which you know bites, or when moving an injured cat. A muzzle must be applied *before* attempting to move or handle the cat. It is difficult, if not impossible, to apply one properly to an already aroused and struggling cat.

Use a long strip of cord, gauze bandage or cloth. Form a loop and slip it over the cat's nose as far as possible. Draw the loop tightly around the nose with the ends under the chin.

MUZZLE

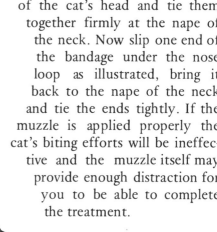

Then bring an end along each side of the cat's head and tie them together firmly at the nape of the neck. Now slip one end of the bandage under the nose loop as illustrated, bring it back to the nape of the neck and tie the ends tightly. If the muzzle is applied properly the cat's biting efforts will be ineffective and the muzzle itself may provide enough distraction for you to be able to complete the treatment.

Wounds and Bandages
Wounds which require repeated cleansing at home are infected traumatic wounds and abscesses (see page 118). These wounds are left open or partially open when treated to allow pus drainage and cleaning. A three percent solution of hydrogen peroxide, which you can buy in drugstores, is suitable for use in such wounds. The best way to use it is described on pages 119 and 121 where you will find more information about wounds, infection and abscesses.

Wounds usually heal most rapidly when left uncovered. In cases where the wound is continually becoming contaminated or when the cat licks at the area so much that they are preventing healing or making it worse it must be protected. Fortunately these occasions are rare involving cats because bandages are more difficult to apply to and to keep on these small animals than on larger ones such as dogs.

A light bandage for a foot can be made by placing an infant or doll stocking over it and taping the sock to the leg with several wraps of adhesive tape applied to the top of the sock and the leg. (Be sure the tape is loose enough to allow circulation to the foot.) This type of wrap leaves most of the sock loose and allows some air circulation. It is best for covering the nails of the rear feet to prevent damage when a cat is scratching at a wound or to protect areas of the foot from licking. Ointments can be applied under such bandages and the sock will keep the medication on the foot and off the carpet.

Bandaging The Foot

SOCK BANDAGE

When cats object to a light weight bandage such as the stocking and repeatedly tear it off, a more substantial foot bandage can be made by covering the whole stocking with tape or by using roll or tubular gauze and adhesive tape. Before applying a substantial bandage, pad the areas between the toes with small pieces of cotton. Depending on the site of the wound, you may want to cover it with a gauze or nonstick pad. Wrap the foot firmly with the gauze, applying several layers vertically as well as around the foot. Follow the gauze with adhesive tape. The long vertical strips not only form the end of the bandage, but help prevent it from wearing through. Try to apply even pressure from the toes to the top of the bandage so normal circulation to the foot is maintained. Don't be too concerned if your first bandage doesn't stay in place; a little practice is required to learn how to apply a bandage to a cat's paw properly so it won't slip off.

TAPE BANDAGE

Flexible wire or electrical tape may be wrapped over the bandage to help prevent your cat from chewing at it and removing it. Usually, however, such measures are not necessary. After a few minutes of vigorous objection, most cats begin to tolerate these artificial coverings. Bandages should be changed at least every third day unless your veterinarian directs you differently.

Abdomen, Back And Neck Bandages

Many-tailed bandages can be made from any rectangular or square piece of clean cloth. These bandages are best used to try to prevent a cat from licking at a wound (e.g., incision following surgery) or to help cover open wounds such as abscesses to prevent drainage from damaging carpeting or furniture. If necessary gauze or cotton padding may be placed between the wound and the bandage. This type of bandage is useful to help you cover an area on the neck, abdomen or back, but don't be surprised if your cat wriggles out of even the best applied one.

"MANY TAILED" BANDAGE

ELIZABETHAN COLLAR

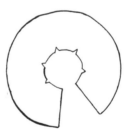
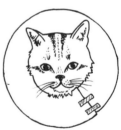

A rare cat will not leave wounds or other irritations alone no matter what bandaging method you try. Also there are occasional wounds, such as those on the head, which cannot be easily protected by bandaging. In these instances you can try an elizabethan collar. Ready-made plastic or cardboard elizabethan collars can be purchased at some pet stores or from some veterinarians. Or you can make one from heavy cardboard as illustrated. This device will prevent most cats from disturbing wounds on their bodies and will prevent the scratching of head or ear wounds. A determined cat can usually wriggle out of even the best applied collar, so be prepared to apply it several times and to administer tranquilizers if recommended by your veterinarian while they are adjusting to the collar. Also many cats cannot or will not eat or drink while wearing an elizabethan collar. Be sure to allow for this by removing the collar when you are home to supervise the cat. Also be sure you know the cause of the problem. A collar will prevent your cat from scratching at their ears, for example, but if they have ear mites, it won't cure them.

Drug Information

General Information

Drugs are identified by their formal *chemical* name, their *generic* name, and their *brand* (proprietary) name. The generic name is usually simplier and easier to remember than the formal chemical name. For example, *acetylsalicylic acid* is the formal chemical name for the drug with the generic name, *aspirin.* If your veterinarian needs to write a prescription, request that they use the generic drug name rather than the brand name, if possible. This allows the pharmacist to give you the same drug usually for less money than the brand name drug would cost.

In general, veterinary drugs are the same as human drugs but less expensive when they are sold under a veterinary label. However, many veterinarians dispense the drugs you need instead of writing prescriptions for you to take to a pharmacy. Although veterinary hospitals make a profit with this practice, for the most part dispensing needed medication this way is a convenience for you and is usually less expensive than purchasing the equivalent medicine at a drugstore. Some companies sell drugs directly to people who are not veterinarians. In some cases the drugs are the same ones veterinarians use. In other cases, however, they are less effective or more likely to be toxic than the drugs a veterinarian would choose. I believe that companies which sell many of these drugs to laymen are interested primarily in profits, not animal health. They usually make few attempts to be sure the drugs are used properly and sometimes fail to warn of possible side effects. Try to avoid such drugs unless recommended by a veterinarian you trust.

All drugs dispensed by a pharmacist or veterinarian should be labeled with the generic or brand name, expiration date, concentration and clear directions for use. This avoids misunderstandings in treatment and helps others who may treat the case later. Since drugs are helpers, not magic potions, your veterinarian should not be secretive about what is being dispensed. Neither should you regard drugs as universal panaceas to be dispensed and used without caution. Caution

210

is particularly important when prescribing medication for cats because they have many idiosyncracies of metabolism which may cause them to react unfavorably to many drugs considered ordinary for use in people or in dogs. Follow your veterinarian's directions for prescription use carefully, and do not use any drug unless it has been recommended by a veterinarian or other *reputable* source for use in your cat. Also keep in mind that drugs are changing all the time. Although I've mentioned some generic drugs safe for use in cats in this book, better drugs may become available before this book is revised. Your veterinarian is usually the best source for the most current information.

Antibiotics

Originally *antibiotics* were chemical substances produced by microscopic organisms that interfere with the growth of other microorganisms. In practice, antibiotics include a large number of substances, many now man made, which are used primarily in the treatment of bacterial infections. Antibiotics are miracle drugs when properly used. They enable us to cure infections that, in the past, would have certainly been fatal. They can, however, be easily misused.

All antibiotics are not effective against all bacteria. A veterinarian's decision to use a particular antibiotic is based on the probable bacteria causing the disease and/or the results of laboratory tests in which the infective organisms are grown and tested for antibiotic sensitivity. If the wrong antibiotic is chosen, there is no beneficial effect. If the proper antibiotic is chosen and given at the correct dosage, growth of the bacteria is stopped or at least controlled sufficiently that the body's own natural defense systems can overcome the infection. If the antibiotic is not given as frequently as prescribed or if the medication is discontinued too soon, forms of bacteria resistant to the antibiotic may multiply, or the infection may recur.

Many people seem to believe that antibiotics are useful in any infectious or febrile disease. This is certainly untrue. A particularly common case where antibiotics may be of no help is the viral infection. *Viruses* exist in body cells and depend on their metabolic processes for reproduction. Since the methods of viral metabolism are unlike those of bacteria, which for the most part survive outside of cells and multiply independently, drugs effective against bacteria are ineffective against viruses. When antibiotics are prescribed for use during viral infection, it is to combat bacteria which invade after the virus has weakened the animal (secondary infection). There are very few drugs available for treatment of viral infections. Since viral reproduction is so intimately tied in with normal cellular function, most drugs found effective against viruses also destroy body cells.

Like other drugs, most antibiotics have potential side effects. Since bacteria are single-celled organisms similar in many ways to individual body cells, antibiotics can sometimes act against body cells in ways similar to the ways they adversely affect bacteria. Among the possible side effects are allergic reactions, toxic effects, alteration of metabolism, and alteration of normal (and beneficial) bacteria inhabiting the body. A good veterinarian will tell you if there are any side effects you should watch for when antibiotics are prescribed. Side effects can be potentiated by the use of outdated drugs, combining antibiotics with certain other drugs, and by certain illnesses.

Indiscriminate use of antibiotics is to be avoided. Use with proper guidance will avoid toxic effects and stem the development of antibiotic-resistant bacteria. Be glad, not disappointed, if your veterinarian feels that the condition can be treated without antibiotics (or other drugs) and sends you away empty-handed. And don't use "leftover" antibiotics unless directed to by your veterinarian. Antibiotics are available over-the-counter as ointments for *topical* (on the body surface) use. Common effective ones contain *bacitracin, neomycin* and/or *polymixin B.* You may wish to instill these into fresh wounds to help prevent infection, but don't let their use give you a false sense of security (see page 119).

Adrenocortical Steroids
Adrenocortical steroids (corticosteroids) include hor-

212

mones produced by the adrenal glands and synthetic drugs similar to these natural substances. This group of drugs has a wide range of actions on the body, among them effects on fat, protein, and carbohydrate metabolism, water balance, salt balance, and cardiovascular and kidney function. They are very important in the individual's ability to resist certain environmental changes and noxious stimuli.

Steroid drugs are commonly used in veterinary medicine for their effects against inflammation. (For example, to give relief from itching due to allergies or other skin diseases.) Because of the remarkable response sometimes possible following administration, some pet owners and some veterinarians are often inclined to misuse these drugs. Keep in mind that steroid drugs are only palliative, relieving but not curing disease unless the condition is caused by deficiency of adrenal gland function. Also keep in mind the fact that steroids are not without side effects. Although they are safe, even lifesaving when used properly, misused they constitute a threat to your cat's health. Avoid preparations containing steroids sold in pet stores and rely on the advice of a good veterinarian regarding the use of steriods in maintaining the health of your cat. Some names of common steroid drugs are *prednisone, prednisolone, cortisone, triamcinolone* and *dexamethasone.* Some have less wide-ranging effects than others.

Drugs You Might Have Around The House

Tranquilizers are drugs which work on the brain in *Tranquilizers* several different ways to achieve desirable behavior in cats. They have legitimate uses in relieving anxiety and producing sedation, and have been helpful in some instances in changing undesirable behavoir patterns. Veterinarians use tranquilizers most often to relieve the anxiety which makes some cats uncooperative when they enter veterinary hospitals, and as preanesthetics. Other common reasons for tranquilizing cats include prolonged confinement (as when traveling), noisy situations (as when being shipped) and sedation to prevent self-trauma (as in wound-licking).

If you can anticipate the need for tranquilization, it is

213

best to discuss the pros and cons with your veterinarian and get a prescription for tranquilizing drugs from them. Cats sometimes react unfavorably to tranquilizers and once tranquilized become less cooperative and more "ferocious" than before. If an unanticipated need arises, two human tranquilizers which can be used in cats are *diazepam* (Vallium®) and *chlorpromazine* (Thorazine®). In such situations call your veterinarian and ask about the advisability of using the drug you have, and ask what the correct dose for your cat should be. Over-the-counter pet tranquilizers contain antihistamines (such as *methapyrilene*) and other drugs (e.g., *scopolamine*) which produce sedation normally thought of as a side effect of their normal uses. In high doses such drugs may produce excitement or may be toxic to cats, and I do not recommend their use. DO NOT use tranquilizers merely for your own convenience; attempt to deal with recurrent problems by training (conditioning your cat to the situation). DO NOT use tranquilizers to sedate your cat following trauma which can produce severe injury (e.g., hit by a car); they can have undesirable side effects on blood pressure in such situations and contribute to shock.

Aspirin   *Aspirin (acetylsalicylic acid)* is a common household drug which is often misused when owners attempt to treat their cats. It relieves fever, mild pain and has some anti-inflammatory effects, but is not a specific cure for any disease. Aspirin relieves fever by acting on the brain to reset the body's "thermostat". The way it brings about its other effects is not known. It is known that aspirin can be very toxic to cats in dosages safe for other animals. Misused it can cause severe signs of illness including vomiting, weakness, lack of appetite, hypersensitivity, blood in the stools, and convulsions. Stomach ulcerations and death have often followed the misuse of aspirin in cats. Since the indications for use of aspirin in cats are few, do not administer aspirin at home. Let your veterinarian decide whether aspirin is necessary and administer it when necessary so overdosage and toxicity do not occur.

214

The use of antiacids is discussed on page 149. *Antiacids*

The use of antidiarrheal drugs (intestinal protectants *Antidiarrheals* and demulcents) is discussed on page 151.

The use of drugs with laxative action is discussed on *Laxatives* page 152.

See page 121 for how to use hydrogen peroxide to clean *Hydrogen* wounds and abscesses. To use it to induce vomiting, see page *Peroxide* 176.

You can try isopropyl alcohol (rubbing alcohol) for *Isopropyl* treatment of inflamed ears; see page 132. *Alcohol*

Breeding and Reproduction

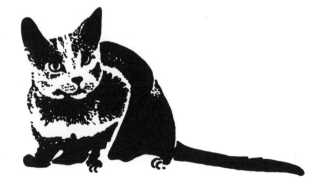

Breeding and Reproduction

General Information

Male (tom) and female (queen) cats usually reach puberty between six and twelve months of age, although some are not mature until fifteen months. The actual onset of sexual maturity and the time of first breeding vary greatly with the individual cat because they are influenced by many factors; among them are climate, nutrition, characteristics of breed and "psychological" maturity. In general, male cats mature physically and breed later than female cats. Although a tomcat may be able to produce sperm and copulate as early as four or five months of age, the actual time he first breeds is dependent on many social factors not associated with physical maturity. A male cat not yet "psychologically mature" and secure in his social position may not breed in spite of the physical ability to do so.

Queens undergo a cyclical physiological rhythm of reproductive function called the *estrous cycle*. This cycle is divided into four stages: *anestrus, proestrus, estrus* and *metestrus*. Of the four stages, however, only two, anestrus and estrus as easily differentiated without laboratory tests.

During anestrus the ovaries are quiescent. This period usually lasts three to four months and usually occurs during the fall and early winter (September or October until January). It may, however, occur any time of the year. The anestrous state can be artifically induced by the *ovario-hysterectomy* of "spaying" operation (see page 221).

219

Anestrus is followed by proestrus, estrus and metestrus which occur sequentially and repeatedly during the spring and summer months. During this period of active sexual cycling *(seasonal polyestrus)* breeding occurs. The *estrus* or "heat" *Signs Of* period, during which the queen is sexually receptive and *Heat* breeding will occur, is usually marked by an obvious change of behavior and voice. The meow becomes lower and very frequent *(calling)*, and the cat usually becomes much more affectionate towards humans, rubbing against them (or inanimate objects) and rolling. Sometimes you may notice increased size of the vulva, but this is extremely variable and is not a reliable sign of heat. If grasped at the nape of the neck with one hand and stroked along with back or genital area with the other, female cats in estrus usually elevate their hindquarters, move their tail to one side and tread (step up and down) with their hindlegs. These same postures occur when a queen

ESTRUS POSTURE accepts a tom for breeding (see page 230).

The changes most often associated with estrus are most easily detected in queens which are kept indoors and not allowed to breed, since the signs may persist nine to ten days in the absence of breeding. Cats with free access to the outdoors or to a tom may pass into and out of heat before you recognize it. Cats are induced ovulators (ovulating in response to breeding) and, if bred, signs of estrus soon pass and pregnancy almost always results. The estrous period in females allowed to breed at will usually has a maximum length of four days. During the breeding season female cats will return to signs of heat about every two or three weeks unless bred or artifically stimulated to ovulate (see page 221). Remember, however, that these time periods are only averages. Each queen has her own normal cycle which, once established, tends to repeat itself.

Preventing Pregnancy

Because the estrous cycle shows a large amount of individual variation and since the onset of heat and breeding can be easily overlooked if your cat has free outdoor access, to prevent pregnancy in an unspayed female you must keep her indoors and isolated from the attentions of unneutered male cats. Although several companies are working on products to prevent pregnancy in cats and dogs, there are no safe and reliable non-surgical methods available now to prevent pregnancy in cats. This means that if you choose to live with an unneutered female cat, you must effectively deal with the recurrent behavioral changes which occur during the breeding season if pregnancy is to be prevented. This can be difficult to do, especially if your cat is one of the more vocal and affectionate breeds (e.g., Siamese). Your veterinarian can help you by providing tranquilizers, which may quiet the behavior to some extent, or they may be able to artifically induce ovulation, thereby reducing the length of the heat period.

Artifical induction of ovulation is achieved by allowing mating with a vasectomized (sterile, see page 227) male cat or by stimulation of the vagina with a glass rod. Such sterile matings produce a state of false pregnancy (see page 231) and can result in a delay of a month or longer before signs of heat occur again. If you desire, your veterinarian can show you the best way to use a glass rod for sterile mating or may be able to put you in touch with an owner of a male cat which has had the vasectomy surgery. Unless your cat is a valuable female for breeding purposes, however, these methods are usually more trouble than they are worth. The best way currently available for preventing pregnancy and eliminating heat behavior is the ovariohysterectomy or spaying operation.

Artificially Induced Ovulation

Many misconceptions surround the spaying surgery. One of the most prevalent is that the spay will cause a female to become fat and lazy. Not so. As stated earlier this surgery induces a permanent condition comparable to the anestrous state. Cats become fat only if they are using fewer calories than they are eating. Inactivity (laziness) usually accompanies

Ovario- hysterectomy Or Spay

excess weight. Fatness can be caused by metabolic abnormalities (e.g., hypothyroidism) but this is rare; it is most often caused by *overfeeding* and is not *caused* by the ovariohysterectomy. Another common misconception is that it is important for a cat to have a litter before being altered (spayed), that having a litter is important to "personality development" or that it "calms them down." In fact, the heat cycle or process of having a litter has no beneficial effect. Although a female cat often has marked changes of personality during estrus, while pregnant and when nursing, once the kittens are gone most females return to their usual anestrous personalities.

The best time to perform the ovariohysterectomy is before the first heat, but most veterinarians recommend not earlier than about five months of age. (It is uncommon for a cat to come into estrus before six months, but it does occur.) The surgery is easiest to perform while the cat is still young (therefore easier on the cat) and it is usually least expensive for you at this time. If you fail to get the surgery performed before heat or breeding occurs, however, don't worry that you will have to have an unwanted litter. Spaying can be easily performed during heat and can also be done during pregnancy although it will probably be more expensive than if performed ealier. *Although there are individual variations,* the procedure for an ovariohysterectomy in most good veterinary hospitals is similiar to the following:

Your veterinarian requests that you withhold food from your cat *at least* eight to twelve hours preceding surgery. This allows time for the stomach to empty, preventing vomiting and aspiration of the vomitus into the trachea and lungs during general anesthesia. Preanesthetic drugs are given to reduce apprehension before surgery and to prepare the body for general anesthesia. Anesthesia is usually induced with a short-acting barbiturate drug even intravenously. Its effects last just long enough to allow the veterinary surgeon to place an *endotracheal tube* into the cat's windpipe (trachea). This airway is the path via which gas anesthetic agents and oxygen are administered to maintain sleep during surgery; it also provides a ready means for resuscitation if any emergency were to arise.

222

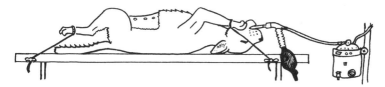

After the cat is sleeping, the abdomen is clipped free of hair, washed with surgical soap and disinfected. The cat is then transferred to the surgery area and placed on the operating table belly up. An assistant stands by to monitor anesthesia, breathing and heart function. The veterinarian, who has been scrubbing their hands and donning sterile clothing and gloves while the cat is prepared for surgery, steps in and places a sterile drape over the patient before surgery begins.

An incision into the abdomen is made at the midline. The length of the incision varies with the size of the cat and the difficulty of the surgery but is usually not more than an inch long. Most veterinarians use a special hook-like instrument to reach into the abdomen and pick up one horn of the uterus as it lies along the body wall. The uterine horn is brought out through the incision and followed to the ovary. Clamps are applied and the blood supply to the ovary is interrupted by *ligatures* (ties placed around blood vessels) or metal vascular clips. The ovary is cut away from its blood supply, which is allowed to return to the abdomen. The other uterine horn and ovary are brought to the incision and treated in the same manner. Then the uterine horns are followed to their point of attachment to the body of the uterus. Its blood supply is interrupted by ties or clips and the uterine body itself is ligated. An incision is made through the uterus to free it, and the horns and ovaries are removed. (Turn to *Anatomy* page 33 if you need to review the structure of the uterus and ovaries.) The inner part of the incision is closed with layers of absorbable suture material or stainless steel; then the skin is *sutured* (stitched) closed. With modern anesthesia, the cat begins to wake up shortly following the last stiches and is ready to go back to an enclosure for final recovery. Most healthy cats are completely themselves one or two days following surgery. In fact, most are feeling so good that is often a chore to try to restrict their exercise.

When you take your female home following surgery, it's a good idea to take her temperature and examine the incision daily even if you are not given specific instructions to do so by your veterinarian. (Good things to do following any surgery.) Fever and/or swelling, redness or discharge at the incision site should alert you to call your veterinarian for advice. Normal feeding should resume forty-eight hours following surgery. Many veterinarians allow you to take your cat home before this time; so if you do, provide meals and water frequently, but in small amounts to avoid stomach upset. Vomiting which occurs more than once or twice, especially if accompanied by inactivity, should again prompt you to call the hospital where the surgery was performed for advice.

Tubal Ligation Some veterinarians and spay clinics perform *tubal ligations* (tying of the fallopian tubes so the ova cannot pass into the uterus). This involves the same type of abdominal entry as an ovariohysterectomy and, although it is effective in preventing pregnancy, I think it has definite disadvantages when compared to an ovariohysterectomy. It does not prevent *pyometra* (see page 162), and it does not prevent signs of heat. If you are *sure* you won't mind living with repeated signs of heat, then you may choose a tubal ligation or, better in terms of health, a *hysterectomy* (removing the uterus but leaving one or both ovaries). Remember, however, that neither prevents the signs of heat. Be sure of your choice or you may be one of the people who change their minds a year or two later and request additional surgery to remove the ovaries.

Accidental Breeding

If your cat was bred accidentally, there are alternatives to having an unwanted litter. If you were planning to have your female spayed, as mentioned before your veterinarian

224

can usually go ahead with the surgery. Usually this is the best and safest step to take. Particularly in the early stages the surgery is not much more difficult than for a female in heat and the fee may be the same. In the later stages of pregnancy the surgery becomes more difficult and the fee increases accordingly.

If you have not yet decided on the question of spaying, and if you can get your cat to a veterinarian soon after breeding (within the first twenty-four hours assuming you *know* your cat has been bred), an injection of an estrogen-like compound followed by oral medication given at home can be used to prevent pregnancy. Compounds used for this purpose work by preventing implantation of the fertilized ova into their "beds" in the uterine wall. These drugs should be used to prevent pregnancy only if you are unwilling to choose another alternative and are willing to accept possible side effects. Their use in cats is not usually recommended by veterinarians since they can be toxic (death can result) and most owners cannot be sure when breeding has actually occurred.

An actual abortion can be performed late in pregnancy if absolutely necessary. Methods similar to those used in humans are not used in cats. Abortions in cats, therefore, consist of *caesarian sections* in which the kittens are removed through uterine and abdominal incisions. This procedure usually results in blood loss, is stressful on the female and is not encouraged by most veterinarians.

Male Birth Control

Castration (removal of the testes) is the traditional method employed for neutering (altering) male cats. Although castration renders a male cat sterile and unable to impregnate a female, this birth control aspect is a minor portion of its importance unless other neighborhood males are also neutered. (One roaming tom can impregnate all the unaltered females in a neighborhood.) The prime significance of castration for most owners of male cats is in the changes of behavior which follow it.

Breeding, fighting, roaming and urine spraying are

Castration

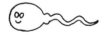

behavioral patterns which are activated when the blood level of testosterone (a hormone secreted by the testes) rises markedly following sexual maturity. Roaming results in encounters between cats—by nature loners—and fighting often results. The wounds and abscesses which follow are not only extremely stressful for the cat but can become very expensive when they occur repeatedly and require veterinary treatment. Urine spraying is a kind of scent-marking behavior associated with territorial identification. The male which is scent marking backs up to the object to be marked, raises his tail and, as the tail quivers, sprays or squirts a small amount of urine onto the vertical surface of the object. Although perfectly normal, this behavior is not acceptable to most cat owners when it is performed around the house. Tomcat urine has a strong and objectionable odor which, together with the stains left from spraying, can be difficult to get rid of.

Benefits Of Castration   Castration before puberty prevents the development of behavioral patterns most often considered objectionable by owners of male cats. Castration later in life, after roaming, fighting and/or spraying has developed, often stops objectional behavior within two weeks, although in some instances improvement takes several months and in a few instances (6-13%) fighting, roaming and/or spraying persists. Castration also prevents the development of "stud tail" (see page 18). And castrated males are generally more affectionate and docile. In other words, a castrated cat is usually a much better pet and companion than his unneutered counterpart.

Castration can be performed by your veterinarian as early as six months of age. Male cats neutered later tend to develop larger bodies and wider heads so if this is a concern to you, you may choose to delay the surgery until undesirable behavioral signs actually develop. The surgery is simple and should be inexpensive. A short-acting general anesthetic is usually administered intravenously. The hair is plucked from the scrotum (see page 31). After disinfection, two incisions are made in the scrotal sac, one over each testicle, and the testes are removed through them after the spermatic duct and the blood supply are interrupted. The

226

incisions are allowed to heal as open wounds. Most veterinarians will send your cat home to recover the same day or within twenty-four hours following surgery. It is a good idea to examine the castration site for signs of infection and to take your cat's temperature daily until the castration wounds are healing well. No special care is necessary later except perhaps to watch your cat's diet. Although castration does not *cause* a cat to become fat, the lower daily calorie needs of an altered male may result in obesity if you allow free choice feeding or overfeed them.

Vasectomy

Vasectomy is rarely performed in male cats. It is the surgical removal of a portion of the *vas deferens* (see page 31) which conducts the sperm from the testes to the urethra. Although vasectomy renders a male cat sterile and unable to impregnate a female, it has no effect on their ability or desire to breed, or other behavior undesirable in a pet, because it does not remove the source of testosterone — the testes. A vasectomy may be useful to the owner of a purebred cattery who desires to keep a sexually active but sterile male available to bring queens out of heat. But since it has no effect on fighting, roaming, urine spraying, grooming or docility, it is not desirable for most house pets. Also, vasectomy is a more difficult, and therefore more expensive, operation than castration.

Cryptorchidism

A *cryptorchid* cat has only one *(monorchid)* or no testicles descended into the scrotum. Males with this condition should not be allowed to breed because the defect is probably inherited. Since both testes are normally present in the scrotum at birth, if they have not descended by six to eight months of age, you should assume that the condition is permanent. Although retained testicles do not produce sperm, they continue to secrete testosterone and must be removed unless you want your pet to continue to act like a tomcat. Retained testicles may be more subject to tumor formation, and although this is a rare problem in cats, it is another reason to be sure that retained testicles are removed. To check the testes, see *Anatomy* page 31.

227

Breeding

Before you decide to breed your cat, ask yourself several questions. The first is: are you sure you will find good homes for the kittens? Except for the most sought after purebred cats, *permanent* good homes are difficult to find. In California alone in 1973 nearly 350,000 cats were destroyed.* It is estimated that eighty to eighty-five percent of all animals entering animal shelters and pounds are killed.* These are not just cats who have strayed from home, but many are pets which have been taken to the pound by owners who know that they will almost certainly be destroyed. They include cats given as unwanted gifts, cute Christmas kittens who have grown into adults and have lost their cuddly charm, cats bought on impulse from pet shop windows, and whole litters intentionally and unintentionally produced for which homes could not be found. Statistics don't include those hundreds of animals which die following abandonment or straying before reaching a shelter or pound, or those killed by humans maliciously or when homes for them could not be found. If you are not *sure* that your kittens won't end up in a pound or pet shop, and if you are not willing to provide a good home for kittens you can't find other homes for, do not allow your cat to breed.

The second question is: do you have a good place to keep the kittens and are you willing to care for them if the mother can't? Even the smallest apartment is usually suitable for raising a litter of kittens since a mother and kittens take up little space, and the mother usually cares for them, at least until around four weeks of age when the kittens begin to consume solid food. But what if the female refuses to care for the kittens or is unable to care for them? Are you ready to assume the responsibility and devote many hours of your time? And what if the mother has difficulty at the time of delivery? You must be willing to plan to be around during delivery to be sure no problems arise, and willing and able to pay veterinary expenses—perhaps for a caesarian delivery—if real difficulties arise.

*1973 California Animal Control Survey, California Humane Council, 4432 Canoga Avenue, Woodland Hills, California 91364

228

Why do you want to breed your cat? Almost everyone is awed by birth and hardly anyone can resist the charm of a kitten, but the cat population cannot afford another litter bred solely so "the kids" or you can watch the birth. If this is the only reason for breeding, it might be best to make arrangements with a dairy, horse farm or established kennel to watch a birth, or to take advantage of films and books available on animal reproduction. If you are breeding for profit, you will find that it can be a fulltime business to produce *quality* purebred cats, care for them properly and still make a profit. Many purebred breeders have cats as a hobby because they know they are likely to break even or take a loss. If you are breeding so the female can "have the experience of being a mother" or so she will "calm down" you are being too anthropomorphic, and possibly falling prey to old wives' tales. I don't think cats can anticipate the experience of having kittens; a few will even neglect their litters to be with their owners. The fact that breeding has no permanent effect on personality has already been discussed. Until the pet animal population reaches a more manageable size, these fascinating and beautiful creatures will continue to experience mistreatment and neglect. Everyone, purebred breeders and pet owners alike, should think these things through seriously before deciding to let their male or female breed and be responsible for the production of even a single litter.

If you decide that it is reasonable to breed your cat you need additional information. Before a female is bred, she should be vaccinated against panleukopenia and rabies (see page 76). Live vaccines should not be given during pregnancy (killed type can be given to a pregnant animal), but the female should be fully protected before breeding so she can pass on a protective level of antibodies to her kittens in the *colostrum* (first milk). Have a fecal sample examined by a veterinarian to be sure that a female to be bred is free from intestinal parasites which compete for nutrients. It is best to avoid breeding most queens on the first heat unless they are definitely full grown. Generally, this means waiting until the cat is at least one year old so she won't have to try

Before Breeding

229

to get enough nutrients to meet both growth requirements and those of pregnancy. No special feeding is necessary before breeding, assuming your cat is already on a balanced diet, but avoid breeding obese females because they will have more difficulties at delivery. If your cat is over five years old at the time you first consider breeding (most unusual for a cat), definitely consider preventing pregnancy. The incidence of difficult births is much higher in animals first delivering in their later years.

The ideal way to insure that breeding will occur is to take the estrus female to the male's home and let breeding occur at will. "Emotional" factors play an important role in determining whether or not a male cat will breed. Often breeding will not occur in an unfamiliar environment; therefore, it is best to take the female to the male. If the male must be brought into the female's home, keep in mind that it may take several days or even several weeks until the male will readily mate, and allow for this when planning breeding schedules. Even when the male feels comfortable and the female is in heat, breeding sometimes will not occur. Female cats in estrus do show preferences for certain males and will sometimes reject one male while readily accepting another.

Breeding Behavior

When placed together, a receptive female (see page 220) and an interested tom will often sniff one another's nose, and the female will rub against the male or roll on the ground. The male moves towards the female's

MATING

back and grabs the skin at the nape of her neck with his teeth. At this time the female will begin treading with her hind-legs, move her tail to one side and strongly curve her back downward. The male slips over the female's back and then moves backward until genital contact occurs. This is followed by several strong and rapid pelvic thrusts resulting in intromission which is quickly followed by ejaculation. Within five to ten seconds after actual breeding has occurred the female usually emits a loud cry, and the male rapidly

230

dismounts and springs away to avoid being scratched by the female. The female usually licks at the vulva, then rolls and rubs on the ground (the afterreaction). If the cats are left together, this series of events may be repeated three to five (or sometimes more) times in an hour.

The female may lose her receptivity to the male (willingness to breed) as early as twelve hours following mating, but, on the average, ovulation occurs twenty-seven hours following breeding. A return to the non-receptive state follows ovulation. After breeding, be sure to confine your cat until you are sure receptivity has passed. If another male is accepted and breeding occurs again before all the ova have been fertilized by the desired father, the litter could have more than a single father.

Determing Pregnancy

About three to four weeks following conception it is often possible for a veterinarian to feel the fetuses in the uterus through the abdominal wall. At this time they are distinct round lumps in the uterus. Later the fetuses are not so distinct, but usually a veterinarian can confirm pregnancy by palpation since cats are small and the abdominal wall is thin. If necessary, an x-ray film taken after five and one-half weeks of pregnancy (when the kittens' bones are ossified) can be used for confirmation of pregnancy and to determine the number of kittens present.

Following a sterile mating which occasionally occurs in cats, false pregnancy (*pseudopregnancy*) may occur. Although signs are not usually marked, lactation may occur and a rare cat may even make a nest and go through a pseudo-labor. False pregnancy usually terminates spontaneously about five weeks after breeding. Estrogen hormones and/or testosterone can be administered by a veterinarian to relieve severe signs of pseudopregnancy. It is best, however, to avoid hormone treatment if possible since estrogen, in particular, can be toxic to cats, and following hormone treatment some cats appear to remain in continual estrus or anestrus. Cats with repeated pseudopregnancies should have an ovariohysterectomy to prevent recurrent signs.

Care During Pregnancy

Pregnancy normally lasts fifty-six to sixty-five days although some normal pregnancies have lasted as long as seventy-one days. Most queens kitten around sixty-three days. Pregnancy increases the protein and caloric requirements of the mother, but if you have been feeding a good quality, well-balanced diet, no major changes in content or calorie supply are necessary during the first three to four weeks. Throughout pregnancy it is extremely important not to overfeed and/or underexercise—to prevent obesity and poor muscle tone which can cause a difficult delivery. In other words, for the most part you will be treating your cat normally during pregnancy.

High quality proteins such as milk products, eggs, and muscle meat should be used to improve the protein quality of your queen's diet throughout pregnancy if you have not offered them before. Kitten replacement formulas (see page 243) may be used as well to insure a high quality diet. Later in pregnancy (after the fourth week) as total calorie requirements increase, expect to offer up to two times the amount of high quality foods necessary before breeding occurred. Although food intake increases, calorie requirements on a *per pound* basis increase only slightly during pregnancy—from about forty to about fifty Calories per pound per day—because the mother is gaining weight (due to the growth of the fetuses) as her food intake increases. Since it is often impossible for a queen to take in all the necessary food in two meals, particularly as the uterus enlarges and begins to compress the abdominal organs, increase the number of feedings throughout pregnancy and lactation or offer food free choice. If you are using high quality commercial products as the basic diet during pregnancy and providing high quality supplements such as meat, eggs and milk products, vitamin-mineral supplements are not necessary. If you are concerned about possible deficiencies, talk to a veterinarian who can supply your cat with a balanced vitamin-mineral supplement.

Most cats restrict their exercise as the time of delivery approaches. If your cat seems too active during the last week of pregnancy, however, you may have to confine her to certain areas of the house where jumping and running can be prevented.

To minimize psychological stress and to prevent your cat from having her kittens in an undesirable place (like the middle of your bed!), accustom her to warm and draft-free delivery area well before the time of delivery. If your 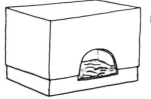 cat has her own bed which she prefers, this is all that is really necessary. Otherwise, provide a maternity box (queening box). The best simple kind is a cardboard box with an opening cut on the side about four or five inches from the bottom. This design provides a convenient entrance and exit for the mother but keeps the kittens from falling out. Introduce the cat to the box daily beginning at least a week before delivery and encourage her to sleep in it by lining it with soft clean towels. If you find that she is not interested but attempts to make a nest in a closet or some other area, you may need to place the nest box there to get her to use it. Since newspapers are easy to remove and discard, it is simplest to line the box with several layers of them at the time of delivery. Clean sheets or towels, however, are just as satisfactory and may be more pleasing to your cat.

Delivery

About five days before the expected date of *parturition* (delivery) you may start taking your cat's temperature morning and evening. At the onset of the *first stage* of labor, the rectal temperature will drop transiently and marketly from the normal of about 101 to 102 to as low as ninety-eight degrees F. At this time, or sometimes earlier, the female will become less active, lose her appetite and seek the nest box. She usually licks frequently at her abdominal and genital areas. Vomiting is a possibility. If you have failed to adjust her to the delivery area, your female may try to nest on your bed, in a closet, or in some other unsuitable spot. Encourage her to remain in the maternity box and stay

233

with her until she becomes comfortable in the area. If she seems particularly distressed about using the box, however, it is best to let her nest where she is most comfortable and try to move the kittens later.

During the *first stage of labor* the female kneads and rearranges the bedding and may even pull hair from her body in her attempt to make a nest. Rapid breathing (sometimes panting) and trembling are often seen, and her pulse rate will increase. Frequent changes of position are made and colostrum may drip from her nipples. Uterine contractions moving the kitten from the uterine horn to the body of the uterus and cervix are occurring during this first stage, which may last twelve to twenty-four hours. A long first stage is particularly characteristic of a first pregnancy. If the signs last twenty-five hours or longer, or your cat seems to pass into the second stage then back to the first, or seems unusually uncomfortable, discuss the matter with your veterinarian before assuming everything is all right.

During the *second stage of labor* you will see forceful straining movements caused by the simultaneous contractions of the abdominal muscles and the diaphragm. At the beginning of this stage you *may* see a small amount of straw-colored or greenish fluid passed at the vulva. This is due to the rupture of the *allantois-chorion* (the protective membrane which covers the kitten) as it passes into the vaginal canal. It may take as long as an hour for a kitten to be delivered once the second stage begins. The female may lie on her side or on her sternum (chest). A rare female will stand and squat as if they were going to have a bowel movement during the most vigorous portions of straining. The *amnion* (membranous sac) enclosing the head of the kitten sometimes appears at the vulva. It may, however, be ruptured before the kitten is delivered. Once the head and paws of the kitten appear, complete delivery should be finished within fifteen minutes—if not, call your veterinarian. The nose and feet of the kitten should not appear and disappear each time the female strains. In the classic birth position the kitten is delivered with its sternum on the vaginal floor, nose first and its front paws along the sides of its face. Nearly half of all

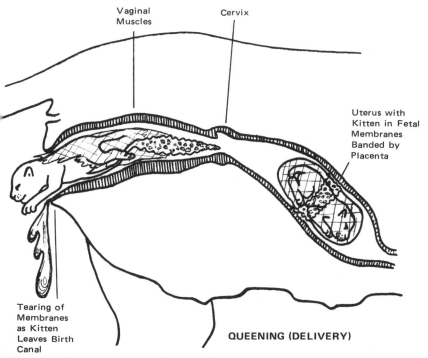

Vaginal Muscles

Cervix

Uterus with Kitten in Fetal Membranes Banded by Placenta

Tearing of Membranes as Kitten Leaves Birth Canal

QUEENING (DELIVERY)

kittens, however, are delivered rear legs first. This usually causes no problem.

As soon as a kitten is delivered, the amnionic sac (amnion) should be broken to allow it to breathe. Cats are usually very good mothers and usually do this immediately, but inexperienced or nervous females may not. If this is the case, you must break the amnion or the kitten will suffocate. However, if the umbilical cord is not broken during delivery, it is not necessary to break it immediately. Significant amounts of blood are found in the placenta, and by allowing the umbilical cord to remain unbroken, you allow time for this blood to pass into the kitten. Normally the mother nips the umbilical cord and breaks it as she cleans and licks the kitten following delivery. If she doesn't do this after about fifteen minutes, a clean piece of thread or unwaxed dental floss should be tied around the cord about one-half to one inch from the body wall. Then cut or break the cord just beyond (distal to) the tie.

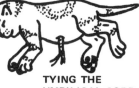

TYING THE UMBILICAL CORD

235

Normally the placenta (afterbirth) is delivered with or just after the kitten. It is a good idea to count the placentas as they are delivered to be sure all are passed. Retained placentas can cause uterine inflammation and infection (see page 162). It is normal, but unnecessary, for the female to eat the placenta following each delivery. It is best to let the queen eat only one or two; the ingestion of too many can cause vomiting and diarrhea.

The time of delivery of the placenta and the period of uterine rest that follows each kitten is the *third stage of labor.* During the rest period the queen usually lies still and tends her kittens though some will get up and take a drink of water. The rest period between kittens varies from about ten to fifteen minutes to several hours. It is not usually more than one to two hours however. Average sized litters for cats range from three to five kittens; average delivery times range from about two to six hours. Normal parturitions, however, may take longer than six hours; some last up to twenty-four or even thirty-six hours.

Difficult Delivery (Dystocia)

Difficult deliveries are usually caused either by obstruction to delivery of the fetus, or by uterine inertia (see page 237). *Dystocia* must usually be treated with the help of a veterinarian. If any of the stages of labor seem abnormally long or if your cat shows signs of excessive discomfort, call your veterinarian.

If you can see a kitten at the vulva, but its delivery seems slow or it appears and disappears, you may be able to help deliver it. Wash your hands and lubricate a finger with a lubricant, like petroleum or K-Y® jelly. Insert your finger into the vaginal canal and move it around the kitten, trying to determine where the head and the front and rear legs are. You may be able to hook a front leg in an abnormal backward position and bring it forward. If the kitten seems fairly normally placed (see illustration page 235), grasp it with a gauze pad, cloth or your fingers and gently pull with each contraction. It is best to try to grasp the kitten around the shoulders to avoid excessive pressure on the head, and it

236

is best to pull downward because the vagina is angled towards the ground. Do not pull on the amnionic sac surrounding the kitten. If the kitten's head just seems too big to fit through the vulva, you can sometimes gently manipulate the edges of the vulva around the head. A veterinarian will sometimes make an incision at the upper part of the vulva to deliver a kitten stuck at the bottom of the birth canal. This cut through the tissue *(episiotomy)* allows the vulvar opening to enlarge. I would advise you not to do this, unless it is impossible to get veterinary help.

If a retained placenta blocks delivery of a kitten, you can often reach it. Grasp it with a gauze pad or cloth and gently but firmly pull until it passes out the vaginal canal. Once an obstruction to delivery is relieved, a female will often have a prolonged rest period before the next kitten is delivered.

Failure of the uterus to contract efficiently *(uterine inertia)* may occur following prolonged straining to deliver a kitten or may be a primary problem, as in the case of an obese or older cat. A form of uterine inertia can be caused by excessive excitement, or by other psychological stresses during delivery. This is why it is important to familiarize your cat with the maternity area well before delivery. It is also why strangers should not be present during delivery unless the cat is extremely calm about them. A labor inhibited by psychogenic stresses can often be helped by having only one or two familiar people remain with the cat during delivery. Rarely, tranquilizers will be necessary.

If no obstruction to delivery is found, your veterinarian may have to administer a drug called *oxytocin* to initiate new uterine contractions. Other drugs may be administered as well. If medical therapy does not initiate proper birth or there is some other problem which cannot be relieved with external manipulations, your veterinarian will want to perform a *caesarian section*—surgery in which the kittens are removed through incisions in the abdomen and uterus. It is usually possible to spay your female (see page 221) at the time of such surgery. Unless the difficult birth is solely attributable to the kittens, it is probably best to have the spay. Mothers who have difficult deliveries tend to repeat themselves. Most queens are able to nurse and care for their kittens normally following caesarian surgery.

Kittens That Won't Breathe

If the queen doesn't break the amnionic sac covering the kitten's head within a minute or two, you should. Then hold the kitten in your hands or wrap it in a towel. Support the head so it doesn't swing freely, then move the whole kitten vigorously in a wide arch from about chest to knee level. At the end of the arc the kitten's nose should point toward the ground. This helps clear excess fluids from the nose and major airways. Other methods to remove excess fluids are to put

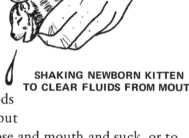

SHAKING NEWBORN KITTEN
TO CLEAR FLUIDS FROM MOUTH

your mouth over the kitten's nose and mouth and suck, or to use an infant ear syringe to suck the fluid from the kitten's mouth and throat. After clearing the airways, rub the face, chest and body of the kitten with a rough towel. If the kitten still does not start to breathe and cry, take in a breath of air, place your mouth over the kitten's nose and mouth and blow gently until you see the chest expand. Remove your mouth and let the kitten exhale, then repeat. Shaking and towel drying even healthy kittens is a good idea if the mother is not interested or is too slow, but this is not absolutely necessary.

Care of the Female Following Delivery

Although for the first two days the queen will stay almost constantly with her kittens, within twenty-four hours of delivery she should leave the nest for short periods of time, move about and be normally interested in eating and

238

drinking. For cats which do not eat or drink·after delivery or which seem abnormally quiet or inactive, as well as those which seem to neglect their kittens, there should be no delay in arranging for examination by a veterinarian. Problems following delivery are too complex to be treated well at home without veterinary consultation.

Shortly after delivery a brownish-red vulvar discharge may be seen, but this should change to clear mucous or no discharge at all within a week following delivery. A bright red, bloody discharge following delivery, a persistent greenish or greenish-black discharge, or any vulvar discharge which is odorous or looks like pus or seems to be present in abnormally large amounts should alert you to take your cat to a veterinarian for a thorough examination. Such abnormal discharges may indicate excessive internal bleeding, retained placenta or kitten and/or uterine infection (see page 162).

If all seems well with the mother, little special treatment is necessary. Keep her indoors following delivery. Heat often occurs within one to four weeks following delivery, and she may become pregnant at this time while still nursing newborn kittens. Since lactation itself is a great stress and the uterus has not had sufficient time to return to its pre-pregnancy condition, breeding should not be allowed at this time. Keeping the queen indoors also avoids exposure to diseases which she could catch or carry home to the fragile nursing kittens. Her diet the first few days following delivery can be the same as that just before. As lactation progresses, however, expect her food intake to increase. A rule of thumb to use is to feed the normal maintenance requirement (about forty Calories per pound per day) *plus* one hundred to one hundred twenty-five Calories per day per pound of kittens. And be sure to continue to feed a high quality, high protein diet since, as in pregnancy, protein requirements for lactation are higher than normal. By the end of lactation a female may be consuming three to four times as much food as she was prior to breeding; in fact, it is almost impossible to overfeed a nursing queen! But despite all "rules of thumb," the best guide to feeding is the appearance of the cat. If she is thin and "worn out" looking her diet may need adjustment.

239

Balanced vitamin-mineral supplements are probably most beneficial when used during lacatation.

Problems Following Parturition

Diarrhea is not uncommonly seen in queens during lactation. Although diarrhea can be a sign of serious illness (see pages 78, 83, 150 and *Index of Signs*), if the cat's temperature is normal and she seems well in all other respects, diarrhea is often a sign of the need for dietary adjustment. The most common cause is that a high enough quality diet is not being fed; i.e., the diet contains too much undigestible material which passes through the gastrointestinal tract unchanged. You may find this problem if the major part of your lactating cat's diet consists of cheap (low quality) commercial foods or dry or semi-moist foods which are comparatively high in fiber content. Dietary changes you can make to alleviate diarrhea in nursing queens are to decrease or eliminate dry or soft-moist foods, be sure canned foods are high quality, and offer highly digestible foods such as cooked eggs, cooked muscle meats and milk products (if they do not normally give your cat diarrhea). Veterinarians can also provide you with high quality, easily digested canned diets. If the stool is extremely watery or if these diet changes do not improve your cat's condition, consult your veterinarian for further help.

Other problems which may affect the female following parturition are infection of the uterus *(acute metritis)*, inflammation of the mammary glands *(mastitis)*, and milk fever *(puerperal tetany)*. These problems are covered in *Diagnostic Medicine* pages 162 and 126 and *Emergency Medicine* page 183.

Care of Kittens Following Delivery

It is a rare queen who needs help caring for her kittens following delivery. The most common problem with kittens following delivery is caused by people who are too anxious to handle the kittens, upsetting the mother and causing her to move them from place to place. Since it is not customary for a veterinarian to examine the queens and kittens immediately

240

after delivery (since problems are uncommon and handling may cause psychological upset), it is wise for a person with whom the queen is familiar to examine the kittens thoroughly about twenty-four hours following delivery to be sure they are free from defects (see page 246). After this, restrict handling of the kittens to about once per day until their eyes are open and they are moving about freely. A normal litter is quiet, and the kittens sleep most of the time they are not nursing. Kittens that cry and squirm continuously should alert you to look for signs of neglect or illness, such as weakness, inability to nurse, diarrhea or lowered body temperature. If you find these or other signs of illness or defect, have the litter examined by a veterinarian, since treating young kittens is difficult.

First time mothers may not have much milk during the initial twenty-four hours following delivery. The first milk is *colostrum*, which is high in antibodies (see page 76) to help protect the kittens from illness during the first few weeks of life. If at all possible, the kittens should suckle the first milk soon after birth, since they are best able to absorb these special proteins through their intestines for only the first twenty-four to thirty-six hours of their lives. Only small amounts are necessary, so don't be alarmed unless the mother's milk supply continues to seem small after the first twenty-four hours. (Test this by looking at the fullness of the mammary glands and squeezing a nipple with a milking action, from near the body to the nipple tip, with your fingers. It should be easy to express a few drops of milk.)

Cats which ignore or actively reject their litters should be examined by a veterinarian, who can sometimes solve the problem by prescribing tranquilizers. In some of these instances, however, nothing helps. In such cases and at times when there is insufficient milk, or if the mother dies, you must take her place.

If it has not been possible for the kittens to suckle the colostrum, your veterinarian may want to administer cat serum as another means to protect the kittens from disease. But discuss this with your veterinarian for each individual situation. Then assume care of the kittens or foster them to another nursing mother. (Nursing cats readily accept new kittens.) Try to cross foster orphan or rejected kittens onto mothers with kittens the same size, or supervise nursing to be sure all are getting sufficient milk.

Kittens which must be separated from a mother must be kept in a warm environment free from drafts because they have difficulty controlling their body temperatures. From birth to about five days of age, the room or box temperature should be eighty-five to ninety degrees F; from about five to twenty days about eighty degrees F. After twenty days the environmental temperature should be lowered gradually to somewhere between seventy and seventy-five degrees F by the fourth week. The best way to provide the proper temperature for orphan kittens, if you don't have a human or poultry incubator, is to use an electric heating pad. Hang the heating pad down one side of the box and onto about one-fourth of the bottom. Then adjust the temperature control to maintain the proper air temperature. By covering only part of the floor you allow the kittens to get away from the heat if necessary. The heating pad and box bottom should be covered with newspaper or cloth which is changed each time it becomes soiled. Most authorities recommend that each kitten be kept in a separate compartment until two or three weeks old to prevent them from sucking each others ears, tails, feet and genitals, but if they are allowed to suckle sufficiently at each nursing period, you will probably find that this is not necessary.

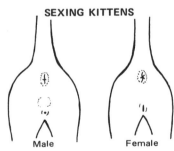

SEXING KITTENS

Male   Female

Research indicates that kittens handled daily are more emotionally stable and resistant to stress. This does not mean, however, that children should handle them without direction or that they should be handled by strangers (who can carry disease). Handling while feeding is sufficient for kittens less than three weeks old. Expect the dried umbilical cord to fall off a normal kitten two or three days following birth. Eyes

242

open around ten to twelve days of age and the ear canals open about two days later. Use the illustration to help you sex the kittens.

Orphan kittens should be fed the formula that most approaches the composition of normal queen's milk. Although you can get by with home formulas made from cows' milk, cat's milk is very high in protein (about twice as much as cow's milk, about five times as much as human milk) and comparatively high in fat, and commercial formulas designed for cats (e.g., KMR®, kitten milk replacers) come much closer to the real thing. These commercial formulas are usually available in pet stores and from some veterinarians, but if they aren't, you can use similar formulas designed for puppies (e.g., Orphalac®, Esbilac®, Havolac®) which are usually readily available. Commercial orphan formulas can be used to supplement feed large litters as well. The best way to determine how much formula each kitten needs is to weigh the kitten and use a table of calorie requirements. The required amount of formula is then divided into three portions fed at eight hour intervals unless the kitten is very small. Kittens weighing less than four ounces may do better with feedings spaced at six hour intervals.

Calories Needed/Pound	Week
190	1
125	2-5
100	5-10

(Example: A four ounce kitten needs ¼ x 190 = 47.5 Calories per day during the first week of life. This is about 1.6 ounces of formula, a little over three tablespoonful, containing 30 Calories per ounce.)

If you supply the proper caloric requirements you do not need to feed most kittens more than three times a day. However, if the kitten cannot take in the required volume at three feedings, the number of feedings must be increased. At each feeding the kitten should eat until just comfortably full—not until the abdomen is tight and distended. A steady weight gain (about 100 to 150 grams per week) and a normal stool are indicators that the kitten is being fed properly.

243

Home Formulas For Orphan Kittens

Evaporated milk	4 oz.	Whole cow's milk	26.5 oz.
Water	4 oz.	Cream (12% fat)	6.5 oz.
Corn Syrup	½ oz.	Egg yolk	1
Halibut liver oil	2 drops	Bone meal	6 gm.
Thiamine hydrochloride	1 mg.	Citric acid	4 gm.
		Vitamin A	2,000 IU
		Vitamin D	500 IU

About 30 Calories per ounce   *About 38 Calories per ounce*

Whole cow's milk	16 oz.
Corn syrup	1 tsp.
Egg yolk	1
Table salt	pinch
Vitamin-mineral supplement as per pkg. or veterinarian's instructions	

About 24 Calories per ounce

All formula is best fed after warming to body temperature (about 100 degrees F). Formula can be administered with an eye dropper, nursing bottle, syringe, or stomach tube. A nursing bottle and nipple are usually easiest and safest in inexperienced hands. The holes in the nipple should be enlarged if the formula does not drop slowly from the nipple when the full bottle is inverted. Be sure the nipple size is suitable for a kitten.

KITTEN NURSING FROM BOTTLE STAND

Hold the kitten on its stomach. Gently separate the lips with your fingers and slip the nipple in. A healthy, hungry kitten will usually suck vigo-rously after tasting the

FEEDING A KITTEN WITH A SYRINGE

If this seems too unnatural wrap the kitten in a towel

milk. Use of a towel will give the kitten something to push

and knead against as if nursing naturally. Weak kittens may have to be held vertically and the formula placed slowly in their mouths with an eyedropper or syringe. DO NOT place a kitten on its back to feed it or squirt liquid rapidly into its mouth. These methods can cause aspiration of the fluid into the lungs, which will be followed by pneumonia. If you wish to use a stomach tube for feeding (the fastest method), ask your veterinarian for a demonstration.

After each feeding the kittens should be stimulated to urinate and defecate. Moisten a cotton swab, tissue or soft cloth with warm water and gently, but vigorously massage the ano-genital area. Nursing kittens' stools are normally firm (not hard) and yellow. If diarrhea develops, the first thing to do is to dilute the formula by about one-half by the addition of boiled water. If this does not help within twenty-four hours, consult a veterinarian. Feeding cow's milk often causes diarrhea because of its high lactose content.

Weaning

Between the ages of three and four weeks you can start to wean most kittens. Place a shallow pan of formula on the floor of their box. At first the kittens will step and fall into it and make a general mess, but soon they will be lapping at it. When this stage is reached, high protein pablum, meat or egg yolk baby food, or commercial cat foods can be added to make a gruel. After they are eating the gruel, the amount of formula can be decreased until they are eating solid food and drinking water. Eggs, cottage cheese, yogurt, and meat may be added to their diet as they become adjusted to eating solid food. Kittens with a natural mother should be allowed to continue nursing during the weaning process until they are eating well-balanced meals of solid food on their own. All changes in feeding should be made gradually to avoid causing digestive upsets.

By five weeks of age the kittens have most of their baby teeth, so that the mother will usually become more and more reluctant to nurse. As the kittens increase their intake of solid food, the mother will gradually reduce her intake of food (or you should) and gradually restrict nursing time.

245

Weaning may be achieved completely this way. But if there is an actual weaning day, offer the queen water but no food, or feed only a small portion of the maintenance diet on that day. Over the following five days gradually increase food back to the normal maintenance level. This procedure helps decrease her milk production.

If milk production does not seem to decrease rapidly enough and the female seems uncomfortable, DO NOT remove milk from the glands. This will only prolong the problem. Cold packs applied to the mammary glands may help, as may camphor oil. If the problem is severe, consult a veterinarian for help.

Umbilical Hernias and Other Defects

Serious birth defects are uncommon in kittens, but each member of the litter should be examined soon after birth and watched as they develop to detect any which may be present. Problems to look for soon after birth include cleft palate (hole in the hard palate, see page 29, so nursing is difficult or impossible), imperforate anus (anus sealed closed by skin so stool is not passed) and umbilical hernia.

A *hernia* is a protrusion of a part of the body or of an organ through an abnormal opening in the surrounding tissues. In an umbilical hernia a portion of fat or internal organs protrude through an incompletely closed umbilical ring. Most umbilical hernias are present at birth, but some may be acquired if the mother chews the umbilical cord too short, or through other careless handling of the cord. Umbilical hernias in kittens are usually small, often get smaller as the kitten ages, and usually do not require surgical repair. If your kittens have large umbilical hernias or hernias you can push into the abdomen with your finger, consult your veterinarian about the necessity of repair.

Problems which are noticed after the first three weeks of age usually consist of abnormalities in the development of walking. Incoordination may result when kittens are infected with the panleukopenia virus while still in the uterus. There are, however, many other causes of locomotor difficulties. If you notice any, a veterinarian should be consulted.

246

Infectious Conjunctivitis (Ophthalmia Neonatorum)

Signs of infection of the conjunctiva are often seen about the time that kittens begin to open their eyes (ten to twelve days). Sticky yellow discharges are present which often seal the eyelids shut until you or the mother cat cleans them, and soon after being cleaned away they return. In some instances the infection is so severe that the lids do not open and severe damage to the eye itself occurs. This type of infectious conjunctivitis of kittens is caused by various bacteria and bacteria-like organisms which are thought to be acquired while the kittens are still in the uterus or soon after birth, from the mother.

If you notice signs of conjunctivitis in your kittens or if their eyes do not open on schedule, early treatment is important to avoid permanent damage to the eyes. The best procedure is to take the whole litter to your veterinarian who can tell you whether actual eye damage is present or likely to occur. If the infection is simple they will provide you with an appropriate antibiotic ointment which you will be instructed to instill into the eyes several times a day after removing the discharges.

You, Your Cat and
Your Veterinarian

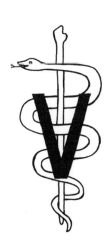

You, Your Cat and Your Veterinarian

Choosing a veterinarian is one of the most important decisions you will have to make concerning your cat's health.

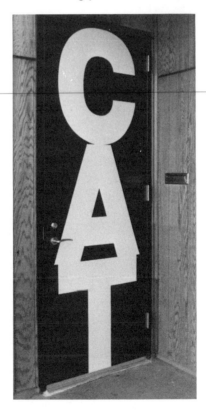

There are bad veterinarians as well as good ones, just as in any profession. I can offer no specific rules for finding the best one for your cat. However, some of the following ideas may help you in your search.

Find a veterinarian you feel comfortable with. No matter how skilled the veterinarian, you cannot make the best use of the services of someone you dislike personally or feel uncomfortable being around.

A good veterinarian explains things thoroughly and in a manner you can understand. There is a shortage of veterinarians in the United States; this puts great demands on their time. Because of this, your veteri-

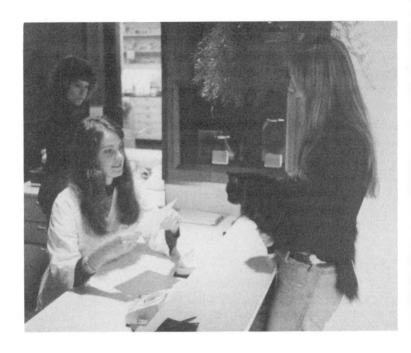

narian may sometimes seem rushed or fail to explain things thoroughly to you. I think this is understandable, but if it happens and you are disturbed about it, let your veterinarian know. There is no need for them to give explanations in totally technical terms either. Medical terminology is more exact, but can be confusing to most cat owners, so problems should be explained in general terms whenever possible. Veterinarians who rely continually on technical language when discussing your cat's health may be on an "ego trip" or trying to "snow" you. Sometimes, though, they are so familiar with medical terms that they forget you aren't. Let your veterinarian know when you are having trouble understanding them, and request a more simple explanation. A good veterinarian will appreciate and heed a polite request.

Good and bad veterinarians exist in all age groups. Don't fall into the trap that an older veterinarian knows more and a younger one less, and vice versa. In general, veterinarians who have been in practice for a while have more experience, but, remember, not everyone learns from experience. A recent

252

graduate often has better knowledge of new techniques available, but may seem clumsy or insecure. Keep these things in mind, and try to evaluate your veterinarian on the quality of care they give your pet. The best veterinarians are continually improving their skills through continuing education as they practice.

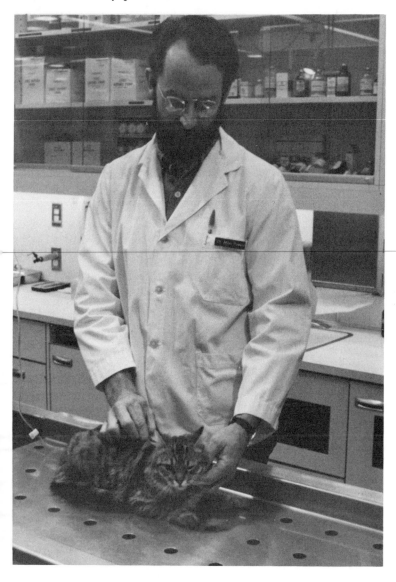

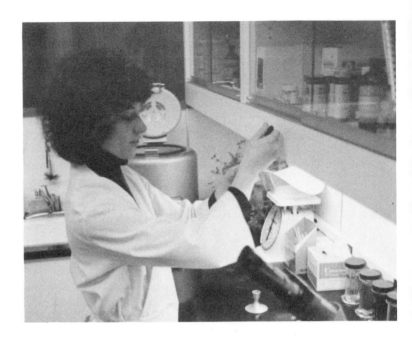

One way to evaluate a new veterinarian is through your first office call. You should see the veterinarian personally, not be required to leave your cat and "check back later" or have lay help take care of the whole problem. The people who handle your pet, both assistants and veterinarians, should seem capable and should use a minimum of restraint on nervous animals unless they have made an attempt to "make friends" without success. A thorough physical examination should be performed and pertinent questions regarding your cat's medical history should be asked. Unless your cat sees the veterinarian extremely frequently, a general physical should always be performed at each visit.

A clean office and new equipment are often indicative of good veterinary care. But don't be misled by a fancy "front room." Most good veterinarians will allow you to see the whole hospital *at a convenient time.* One who won't may have something to hide. Some veterinarians have fancy equipment but don't use it or use it improperly. Veterinarians in small towns or rural areas may not have enough demand to necessitate expensive specialized equipment in their offices. Again, try to judge your veterinarian on the kind of medicine practiced, not on appearances.

It is as difficult to judge a veterinarian by their fees as it is according to the kind of equipment in their office. What is a reasonable fee varies with geographical area and type of practice. In general, it is "fair" to expect to pay more for veterinary services at hospitals where the latest equipment and specialized services are available, since it costs the veterinarian more to maintain such services. (Remember, most veterinarians, unlike physicians, don't have large central hospitals for patients who need special care, and so must maintain their own.) If you are concerned about the fee, be sure to ask your veterinarian about it if they don't bring up the matter first.

Veterinarians who don't maintain specialized equipment must refer some of their cases. A good veterinarian recognizes their own limitations. Veterinarians who won't make referrals when requested may be trying to hide their own inadequacies.

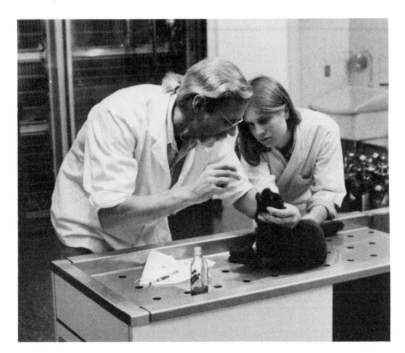

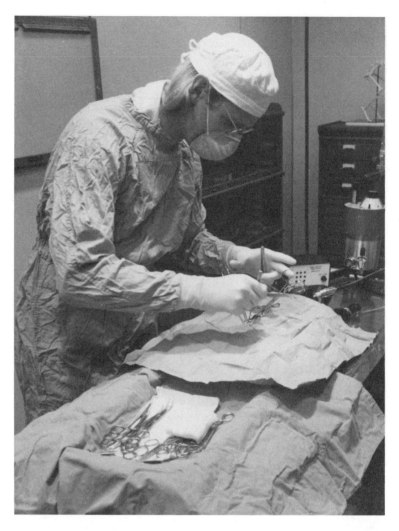

Choose a veterinary clinic which provides emergency service or will be able to refer you to emergency care when necessary. Some communities have central emergency services which work closely with the local veterinarians; others do not. Find out what your veterinarian or the community provides while your cat is healthy so you won't waste precious time when a true emergency arises.

Once you have found a veterinarian who seems capable and interested in providing your pet with good health care you can do even more do assure that your cat is treated well. Like other people, veterinarians are inclined to provide the best service to people who are nice to them ("good" clients). Since veterinarians are people, and as such aren't infallible or tireless, they appreciate consideration on your part. If you keep a few simple courtesies in mind and try to practice them, these signs of appreciation will make most veterinarians respond with their best efforts.

If your veterinarian takes appointments, try to be on time. This helps keep the veterinarian on schedule and helps prevent an extra long wait for others. Avoid "dropping in" without an appointment; call ahead if you have a sick pet and cannot wait another day. Never drop in for routine preventive care such as vaccination or deworming unless your veterinarian chooses not to use an appointment system. And when you do come in be sure to bring your cat in a carrier or on a leash to prevent mishaps and disturbances in the waiting room.

Avoid dropping your cat off for care unless your veterinarian specifically directs you to. Most people would never consider dropping their child off at the pediatrician's, but many seem to expect that veterinarians should provide "one hour, one stop" service and get good results. Your cat usually receives better care if you discuss the problem with your veterinarian as the examination is performed. If your animal is very sick and it is impossible for you to wait for an office call, call ahead and discuss the problem with the veterinarian first. They may be able to advise you on home treatment, and, at least, be able to deal with the problem more calmly than if you show up in a rush hoping to leave your pet with them at the last minute.

Do not disturb your veterinarian at night, on holidays or during their other time off for non-emergency matters. If you have any doubts about the emergency status of an illness, call, but don't call at these times just for general information.

Don't expect your veterinarian to make a diagosis over the phone, or solely on the basis of a physical examination. And don't expect the veterinary hospital to be a drug store, supplying drugs on demand. Competent veterinarians

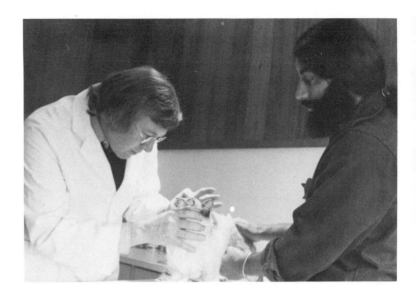

interested in your cat's health want to examine your pet and may require laboratory tests before prescribing drugs or making a diagnosis no matter how sure you are of the problem. They do this not to "hassle" you, but to protect your cat as well as themselves. Don't feel that you can't ever call your veterinarian for advice, however. Just be prepared with some solid facts. If you can tell your veterinarian whether or not your cat has a fever, what the basic signs of their illness or injury are, and how long the signs have been present, they will probably be willing to give you some help over the telephone in spite of a busy schedule. If you can't supply such information, though, don't be surprised if you are told that it is impossible to help you over the telephone.

Don't let signs persist for several days without or in spite of home care before consulting a veterinarian. It is extremely frustrating for a veterinarian to see an animal die of an illness which could have been treated successfully if professional care had begun sooner. And, once you have consulted a veterinarian, please follow their directions. It is quite irritating to have someone complain that a treatment didn't work only to find out later that the medication was not used or used improperly. If you are having trouble

258

following their instructions, notify your veterinarian, but don't stop treatment without their advice.

Learn to use your veterinarian as a resource for your animal's health. Know that help is there when you need it, but use this book, your patience and your common sense to take most of the responsibility for your cat's health. This book is intended as a tool to help you determine the limits of your responsibility and when you should draw on the veterinarian's resources. By using it this way you will be practicing preventive medicine and may forestall illness and extra medical costs before they develop. Remember your relationship to your cat, and your moods and your attitude toward their health and well-being are vital factors in their health care and in the effectiveness of your veterinarian. If you can temper your concern for your animal with an intuitive understanding of them and with the knowledge you have gained about their health care from this book, you will avoid needless emotional upset and promote the growth of the three-way relationship of health—you, your cat and your veterinarian.

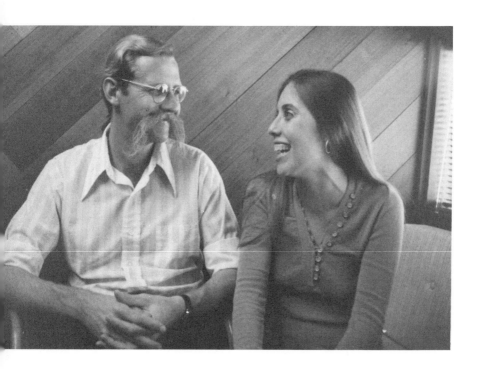

Since I had planned to be a veterinarian from the time I learned that there were "doctors for animals," but never considered writing until recently, I find myself somewhat surprised, as well as happy and relieved, to be finishing another book. Of course, without a great deal of help neither the Well Dog Book *nor* The Well Cat Book *could have been written. Don Gerrard is particularly important since he first suggested that I try to write a new kind of book about cat and dog care, and provided important criticism and a lot of encouragement. Tom Reed, a good friend and a veterinarian also, deserves very special thanks for all the time and hard work he gave to illustrate both books. And Diane and George Ahlgren, Nancy Ehrlich, Michael Floyd, Jay Fuller, and Madeline Reed all helped by looking over the manuscript.*

Writing at times has been a real chore, but the effort will be rewarded if you find this book useful. Please write to me at 1550 Solano Avenue, Albany, California 97406 *and let me know how you feel about it. Although I can't answer specific questions about veterinary problems, your thoughts about the book, both pro and con, would be helpful to me. May your animals be well.*

For those of you who own dogs, this book's companion volume, The Well Dog Book, *is available from Random House/Bookworks.*

Terri McGinnis

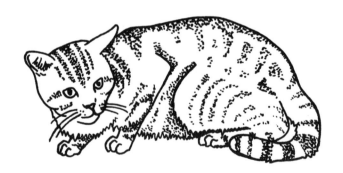

General Index

General Index

266

F

Gums, care of 57–58
    inflammation of (gingivitis) 56, 57–58, 134
    normal appearance 27
    pale 27
    receding 58
    red 58, 134

Hairballs 150

Hair, care of 50–53
    kinds of 21
    loss of (including shedding) 17, 21, 97, 101, 122, 124
    mats in 52
    normal appearance 17, 21
    oil in 52
    paint in 52
    tar in 52

Head mites 101

Head shaking 100, 132

Head tilt 100, 132

Hearing, loss of 185
    test for 185

Heart, anatomy of 36
    disease 188–189
    external massage 174–175
    failure 188
    how to examine 36–37
    murmur 189
    rate 37
    worms 94

Heat (see Estrus)

Heat stress (prostration, stroke) 182

Hemobartonella 164

Hematoma 133

Hemostasis 170–171

Hernia, definition of 246
    diaphragmatic 172–173
    umbilical 127, 246

Hit by car 171–172

Hives 180

Home medical care 191–215

Hookworms 91–92

Hormones 39

273

274

R

275

T

Vulva, normal appearance 33–34
　　discharge from 34
　　swelling of 220

Water, daily need 61, 110
　　during illness 110, 198–199
　　during traveling 75
　　excessive drinking 156, 162, 187

Weaning 245–246

Weight reduction, how to achieve 154–155

Whipworms 93

Whiskers 21

Worms (see Parasites, internal)

Wound, healing 118
　　home treatment 119, 121, 212
　　infection 119–121

W